dietary fats and oils
in human nutrition

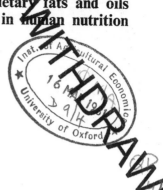

dietary fats and oils in human nutrition

Report of an Expert Consultation

jointly organized by

the Food and Agriculture Organization of the United Nations

and

the World Health Organization

held in Rome, 21–30 September 1977

FOOD AND AGRICULTURE ORGANIZATION OF THE UNITED NATIONS

Rome, 1980

First published 1977
Reprinted (with corrections) 1978

P-86

ISBN 92-5-100802-7

TABLE OF CONTENTS

v

LIST OF ILLUSTRATIONS

LIST OF TABLES

Joint FAO/WHO Expert Consultation
The Role of Dietary Fats and Oils in Human Nutrition

Rome, 21–30 September 1977

A Joint FAO/WHO Expert Consultation on the Role of Dietary Fats and Oils in Human Nutrition was held in Rome 21–30 September 1977. The meeting was opened by Dr. E.M. DeMaeyer of the World Health Organization, Geneva, who expressed the appreciation of FAO and WHO to the participants.

Members

Dr K.T. ACHAYA, Executive Director, Protein Foods and Nutrition Development Association of India, Bombay, India

Dr R.G. ACKMAN, Halifax Laboratory, Fisheries Canada, Halifax, Nova Scotia, Canada

Dr E. AAES-JØRGENSEN, Department of Biochemistry, Royal Danish School of Pharmacy, Copenhagen, Denmark

Dr J.G. BIERI, National Institute of Arthritis, Metabolism and Digestive Diseases, National Institute of Health, Bethesda, Maryland, USA

Dr R. BLOMSTRAND, Professor, Karolinska Institutet, Department of Clinical Chemistry, Huddinge University Hospital, Huddinge, Sweden

Dr M.A. CRAWFORD, Department of Biochemistry, Nuffield Laboratories of Comparative Medicine, The Zoological Society of London, Regents Park, London, UK (*Rapporteur*)

Dr C. GALLI, Institute of Pharmacology and Pharmacognosy, University of Milan, Milan, Italy

Dr F. GRANDE, Instituto de Bioquímica y Nutrición, Fundación F. Cuenca Villoro, Gascón de Cotor, Zaragoza, Spain

Dr A.G. HASSAM, Department of Biochemistry, Nuffield Laboratories of Comparative Medicine, The Zoological Society of London, Regents Park, London, UK

Dr R.T. HOLMAN, The Hormel Institute, University of Minnesota, Austin, Minnesota, USA

Dr Joyce BEARE-ROGERS, Nutrition Research Division, Bureau of Nutritional Sciences, Health Protection Branch, Department of Health and National Welfare, Ottawa, Canada

Dr J.F. MEAD, University of California, Laboratory of Nuclear Medicine and Radiation Biology, Los Angeles, California, USA (*Chairman*)

Dr K.R. NORUM, Institute for Nutrition Research, School of Medicine, University of Oslo, Oslo, Norway

Dr A.M. O'DONNELL, Centro de Estudios sobre Nutrición Infantil, Buenos Aires, Argentina

Dr S.G. SRIKANTIA, Director, National Institute of Nutrition, Hyderabad, India

Dr H. SVAAR, Assistant Professor, Department of Pathology, Ulleväl Hospital, Oslo, Norway

Dr A. VALYASEVI, Department of Pediatrics, Faculty of Medicine, Ramathibodi Hospital, Bangkok, Thailand

Dr A.J. VERGROESEN, Unilever Research, Vlaardingen-Duiven, the Netherlands (*Vice-Chairman*)

Dr F.E. VITERI, Chief, Division of Human Nutrition and Biology, Institute of Nutrition of Central America and Panama, Guatemala City, Guatemala

Representatives of other organizations

Dr F. FIDANZA, Permanent Representative of IUNS at FAO, Università degli Studi di Perugia, Dipartimento di Scienza e Tecnologia, Istituto di Scienza dell'Alimentazione, Perugia, Italy

Mr A.W. HUBBARD, Chairman, Codex Committee on Fats and Oils, Ministry of Agriculture, Fisheries and Food, London, UK

Dr L.J. TEPLY, Senior Nutritionist, Office of the Executive Director, United Nations Children's Fund, New York, USA

Secretariat

Dr D.G. CHAPMAN, Scientist, Food Safety Programme, WHO, Geneva, Switzerland (*Joint-Secretary*)

Dr E.M. DeMaeyer, Medical Officer, Nutrition, WHO, Geneva, Switzerland (*Joint-Secretary*)

Mrs B. Dix, Food Standards Officer, Food Policy and Nutrition Division, FAO, Rome, Italy (*Joint-Secretary*)

Mr G.O. Kermode, Officer-in-charge, Food Policy and Nutrition Division, FAO, Rome, Italy

Dr P. Lunven, Chief, Food and Nutrition Assessment Service, Food Policy and Nutrition Division, FAO, Rome, Italy

Dr J. Périssé, Senior Officer, Food and Nutrition Assessment Service, Food Policy and Nutrition Division, FAO, Rome, Italy

Dr N. Rao Maturu, Nutrition Officer, Food and Nutrition Assessment Service, Food Policy and Nutrition Division, FAO, Rome, Italy (*Joint-Secretary*)

INTRODUCTION

There are in the world millions of people whose health suffers because of an insufficiency of the right kinds of food. By contrast, among prosperous people diseases associated with dietary excesses are common. The principal nutritional problem of the developing countries appears to be a deficit of dietary energy, whereas that of developed countries is overconsumption. Furthermore, the contrast in fat intakes is very great. The problem of dietary fat in human nutrition is controversial and complex, and it is, in fact, one of the most important questions yet faced by nutritionists.

FAO and WHO are concerned about the implications of dietary fats in human nutrition because of the positive contribution fats might make to the health and performance of many people and nations, and because of the possible adverse effect of certain fats on atherosclerosis and on obesity and its complications. During the last decade there have been significant advances in knowledge of the nutritional value and physiological effects of different fats. Some of these advances may lead to a revision of current views about the quality of dietary fat.

There are two general considerations: firstly, the importance of fats in food and, secondly, the safety aspects.

Dietary fat is important for five reasons:

(*i*)   as a source of energy;

(*ii*)   for cell structure and membrane functions;

(*iii*)   as a source of essential fatty acids for cell structures and prostaglandin synthesis;

(*iv*)   as a vehicle for oil-soluble vitamins;

(*v*)   for control of blood lipids.

In addition, fat contributes to the palatability of food and is thus important in cooking and food processing.

In considering the safety of fats, a major issue that remains to be resolved is that of the health implications of the brassica-derived oils and partially hydrogenated marine oils. Guidelines regarding the use of such oils and fats for human consumption are urgently needed.

Finally, it is important to establish to what extent crop and animal management affects the nutritional quality of the food eaten.

This publication is a synthesis of the papers presented and the subsequent discussion on them. It attempts to record the current status of knowledge of dietary fats and oils in human nutrition.

1. DEFINITIONS

The definitions used follow those employed in previous FAO/WHO reports, the 1973 report on energy and protein requirements (11) being used as a reference. Because of the specialized nature of lipid biochemistry and nutrition, the following additional information is presented.

Fats and oils

This group of water-insoluble organic substances predominantly consists of triglycerides — i.e., glyceryl esters of fatty acids. Fats are distinguished from oils only by their different melting points: fats are solid and oils liquid at room temperature; however, the general term "fats" is commonly used to refer to the whole group and is synonymous with "lipids."

Classification of fats

Although fats constitute a diverse group of substances, they can be roughly divided into two classes:

(1) *Neutral* fats, which include the triglycerides, cholesterol, other sterols and isoprenoid groups with their esters (vitamins A, D, E and K also fall into this category).

(2)*Amphiphilic* fats, which consist of the phospholipids, the principal members being the choline phosphoglycerides (lecithins), ethanol-amine, serine and inositol phosphoglycerides, together with the sphingo lipids such as sphingomyelin. The amphiphilic group possesses the property of forming bilayers. Because part of the molecule (the phosphate ester) is strongly polar (miscible with water) and the aliphatic part is nonpolar, the phospholipids have the property of orienting on the surface of a large molecule, on an aqueous surface or on an interface between two immiscible layers. It is this property which is thought to play an important part in their biological role in the formation of cell membranes and in their industrial use as surfactants or emulsifiers.

3

Broadly speaking, this chemical classification follows the *biological functions* of the two separate groups of fats in the body:

(*1*) *Storage* fats, mainly triglycerides, which are accumulated in specific depots in the tissues of plants and animals. These fats are the most important energy reserves of the body, and in animals they are also a source of essential nutrients. The composition of the fatty acids in these triglycerides is related to the diet.

(*2*) *Structural* fats, mainly consisting of phospholipids and cholesterol. Quantitatively these are the second most important structural group in all soft tissues of the body and are present in unusually high concentrations in the brain. The fatty acid component of the phospholipids is of crucial importance to their properties and function in biological membranes. The composition of the fatty acids in the phosphoglycerides in general exhibits a tissue and species specificity. Although they are subject to dietary alteration, extreme conditions are needed to change their composition appreciably.

The basic structures of the main group of the fats are shown below:

GLYCEROL   TRIGLYCERIDE   PHOSPHOLIPID
(e.g., choline phosphoglyceride)

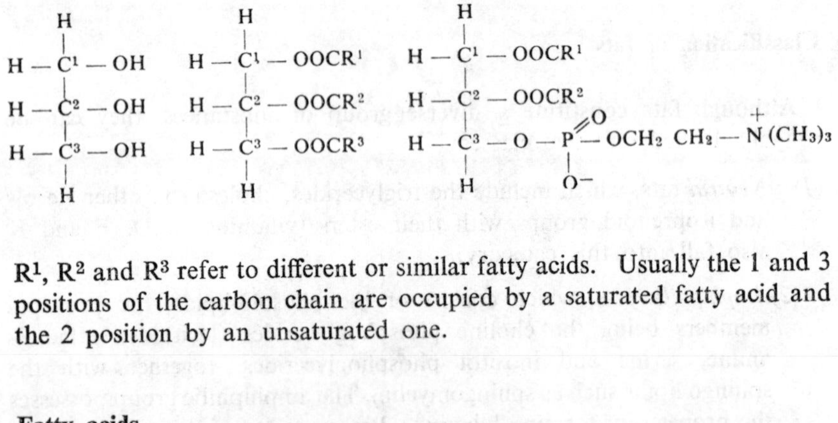

R^1, R^2 and R^3 refer to different or similar fatty acids. Usually the 1 and 3 positions of the carbon chain are occupied by a saturated fatty acid and the 2 position by an unsaturated one.

Fatty acids

The principal fatty acids of relevance to this report are mostly straight chain aliphatic monocarboxylic acids with an even number of carbon atoms. Common names and the modified Geneva names of the International Union of Pure and Applied Chemistry (IUPAC) are mostly used for fatty acids. For example: palmitic acid $CH_3(CH_2)_{14}COOH$ is systematically called hexadecanoic acid; stearic acid $CH_3(CH_2)_{16}COOH$

4

is octadecanoic acid; oleic acid $CH_3(CH_2)_7CH=CH(CH_2)_7COOH$ is octadecenoic acid. The fatty acids are mostly found in triglycerides and phosphoglycerides, and some are esterified with cholesterol.

In *saturated* fatty acids all carbon atoms are joined by single bonds and, with the exception of the carboxyl group, all other valency positions are occupied by hydrogen.

In *monounsaturated* fatty acids two adjacent carbon atoms are joined by a double bond. Here, *stereochemical isomerization* can occur because the sections of the molecule on any side of the double bond can lie either on the same (*cis*) or the opposite (*trans*) side of the bond.

cis   trans

Because the double bond fixes the relative positions of the other two sections of the molecule, the cis and trans isomers have different biological properties. Most naturally occurring isomers have the cis configuration. Positional isomers may also occur because the double bond may be variously located within the molecule.

In *polyunsaturated* fatty acids there is more than one double bond. The term polyunsaturated fatty acids covers a wide range of acids of 18, 20 and 22 carbon chain length with two to six methylene-interrupted double bonds. Unless otherwise stated, the double bond sequence is methylene-interrupted and all double bonds have the cis configuration. The fatty acids mentioned in this report are listed with synonyms and abbreviations in Table 1. The diagrammatic representation of fatty acids is shown in Figure 1.

Essential fatty acids

Linoleic (18:2, *n*–6) and α-linolenic (18:3, *n*–3) acids are required for the normal growth and function of all tissues. They have double bonds positioned at six carbons (*n*–6) and three carbons (*n*–3) from the methyl end of the molecule. Animals, including man, cannot insert double bonds in the *n*–6 and *n*–3 positions and cannot synthesize either of the two. However, animals can add more double bonds to the parent essential fatty acid (EFA) by introducing them between the original double bonds

5

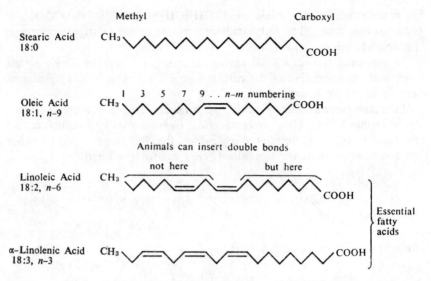

FIGURE 1. Diagrammatic representation of the fatty acids.

and the carboxyl group; at the same time, the carbon chain length is extended at the carboxyl end by further desaturation. This metabolic process produces the long-chain derivatives of 20 and 22 carbon chain length with 3, 4, 5 and 6 double bonds (Table 1). The result is two families (the n–6 and n–3 families) of essential fatty acids which are required for cell structures and prostaglandin synthesis.

The 20 and 22 carbon chain length fatty acids with 3, 4, 5 and 6 double bonds derived from linoleic (18:2, n–6) and α-linolenic (18:3, n–3) acids are referred to as the *long-chain essential fatty acids;* in practice the two most important are arachidonic (20:4, n–6) and docosahexaenoic (22:6, n–3) acids.

Visible and invisible fats

No all-embracing definition yet exists that will satisfy the pathologists, nutritionists and technologists who are professionally concerned with fats. For the purpose of this report, the terms *visible* and *invisible* (as used in food processing) are employed to divide fats into separated and unseparated. Visible fats are those which have been separated from animal tissues, milk, oilseeds, nuts or other vegetable sources; they are used to produce shortening, margarine, salad oils, butter, etc. Invisible

TABLE 1. – NOMENCLATURE OF FATTY ACIDS USED IN THE REPORT

Common name	Synonym [1]	Abbreviation [2]
capric	decanoic	10:0
lauric	dodecanoic	12:0
myristic	tetradecanoic	14:0
palmitic	hexadecanoic	16:0
stearic	octadecanoic	18:0
oleic	9-octadecenoic	18:1, n–9
arachidic	eicosanoic	20:0
gadoleic	11-eicosenoic	20:1, n–9
behenic	docosanoic	22:0
erucic	13-docosenoic	22:1, n–9
brassidic	trans-13-docosenoic	trans 22:1, n–9
cetoleic	11-docosenoic	22:1, n–11
lignoceric	tetracosanoic	24:0
nervonic	15-tetracosenoic	24:1, n–9
linoleic	9, 12-octadecadienoic	18:2, n–6
γ-linolenic	6, 9, 12-octadecatrienoic	18:3, n–6
α-linolenic	9, 12, 15-octadecatrienoic	18:3, n–3
dihomo-γ-linolenic	8, 11, 14-eicosatrienoic	20:3, n–6
	5, 8, 11-eicosatrienoic	20:3, n–9
arachidonic	5, 8, 11, 14-eicosatetraenoic	20:4, n–6
	5, 8, 11, 14, 17-eicosapentaenoic	20:5, n–3
	7, 10, 13, 16-docosatetraenoic	22:4, n–6
	4, 7, 10, 13, 16-docosapentaenoic	22:5, n–6
	7, 10, 13, 16, 19-docosapentaenoic	22:5, n–3
	4, 7, 10, 13, 16, 19-docosahexaenoic	22:6, n–3

[1] Double bonds numbered from the carboxyl end. – [2] Fatty acid formulae are abbreviated in the form x:y, n–m where x = number of carbon atoms in the molecule, y = number of double bonds, and m = position of the first double bond numbered from the methyl end. Thus, palmitic acid is 16:0 and linoleic acid 18:2, n–6. Where the n–m specification of the double bond sequence is omitted, then either the position is not known or, where isomers are present, the whole group is being referred to. For example, 22:1 would refer to an undefined mixture of isomers which could include 22:1, n–9, n–11 and trans 22:1, n–9.

fats are those which have not been separated from their original source and are therefore consumed as part of the tissues in the diet — principally as meat, fish, poultry, dairy products, cereals, pulses, nuts and vegetables.

The difficulty with this definition is that invisible fats in fatty meats are considered in the same context as invisible fats in foods of vegetable origin and fish. As the awareness of the different types of fats in nutrition grows, these definitions may need to be reconsidered.

Units of energy

Many nutritionists are accustomed to expressing dietary energy in kilocalories. In the International System of Units (SI) the unit of force is the newton, which accelerates 1 kg by 1 m/s². The unit of energy is the joule (J), which is the energy expended when 1 kg is moved 1 m by 1 newton. In this report, energy values are expressed both in joules and calories.

$$
\begin{aligned}
1 \text{ kilocalorie (kcal)} &= 4.184 \text{ kilojoules (kJ)} \\
1\,000 \text{ kilocalories (kcal)} &= 4\,184 \text{ kilojoules (kJ)} \\
&= 4.184 \text{ megajoules (MJ)}
\end{aligned}
$$

The energy value of fat is taken as equivalent to 9 kcal (37.7 kJ)/g, of protein as 4 kcal (16.7 kJ) and of carbohydrate as either 4.2 kcal (17.6 kJ) or 3.75 (15.7 kJ)/g, depending on whether the carbohydrate is expressed as polysaccharide or monosaccharide [in practice, a value of 4 kcal (16.7 kJ)/g is used for carbohydrate].

2. FAT AS A SOURCE OF ENERGY

Introduction

Man derives his energy from the three major nutrients: protein, fat and carbohydrate. Of these energy sources, fat has the highest available energy value, 9 kcal (37.7 kJ)/g, as compared with 4 kcal (16.7 kJ)/g for protein and carbohydrate. Diets of most countries provide an average of about 11% calories from protein, although isolated extremes of 6% to 30% have been recorded (1).

In most parts of the world the nonprotein dietary energy ranges from 80% to 90% of the total and comes from fat and carbohydrate. In some communities alcohol may make a significant contribution to the energy intake. Depending upon the food supply and the family income, the intake of fat is found to vary widely between different countries and also within the same country. In the developed countries average energy intakes from dietary fat currently range from 35 to 45 energy %; however, high fat intakes (>30 energy %) are not found solely in those countries.

In many developing countries, intakes of 10 to 20 energy % of fat or less are common and have been habitual for many generations (2, 3). Thus, on a global basis, there could be an approximately sixfold difference in the fraction of energy derived from fat by various populations.

In addition to the differences in amounts of fat consumed, there are wide variations in the sources of fat. In the past, fat sources have been categorized as animal or vegetable, but it is now known that this classification is too broad and must be refined to give a better description of the metabolic effects different fats may produce.

Dietary fats (lipids) are mainly triglycerides composed of fatty acids of varying chain length which may be saturated, monounsaturated or polyunsaturated. The relative proportions of saturated and polyunsaturated fatty acids in the diet may be of primary importance in determining their nutritional implications. In diets very low in fat, phospholipids may constitute a relatively high proportion of the fat as they are a component of all vegetable and animal cells. In some parts of the world, especially in Asia, dietary fat is predominantly of vegetable origin; elsewhere, animal fats may constitute one half to two thirds of the dietary fat. Thus a wide variety of fats and oils with differing physical and chemical properties and fatty acid composition are consumed. With a few exceptions, human metabolism can effectively use all of these fats for energy. The fatty acid content of some selected foods is given in Appendix 1.

Functions of dietary fat

Dietary fat is thought to be an obligatory nutrient only as a source of essential fatty acids; nevertheless, it has several desirable, nonobligatory nutritional properties. Its physical characteristics impart a satisfying texture to foods that increases palatability for many people and may contribute to the acceptance of food. Fat also acts as a vehicle for some of the fat-soluble vitamins. Thus dairy fats contain significant amounts of vitamin A (retinol) and D, as do some marine oils. Almost all vegetable oils contain vitamin E and are the richest source of this vitamin in many diets. A few oils (e.g., red palm oil) contain substantial amounts of carotenoids (pro-vitamin A), which can also be found in many vegetables and fruits. Rendered animal fat is a negligible source of fat-soluble vitamins, but invisible fat in meat may have small amounts of vitamin A.

The degree to which the amount of dietary fat affects the utilization of fat-soluble vitamins has not been thoroughly studied in man. For pro-vitamin A, the addition of olive oil to diets with a very low energy % as fat was found to improve utilization, as determined by blood levels (4). There is little or no evidence that within the range of human fat intake the amount of dietary fat significantly affects the availability of preformed vitamin A (retinol) or of vitamins D, E and K.

Although natural fats contain many desirable trace components such as flavours and vitamins, in recent years they have, like other food components, become the vehicle for undesirable fat-soluble compounds. The most common of these compounds are pesticides and other agricultural chemicals, but contamination with industrial chemicals also occurs.

Physiological effects and utilization of dietary fats

Different populations appear to subsist in a good state of health on widely different fat intakes, not only amounts but also types. On the other hand, as societies become more affluent, they tend also to become less physically active, so that a previously satisfactory diet with respect to energy and fat can become a health hazard, leading to obesity. In most developed countries a significant percentage of the population has

10

high blood lipid levels, which are considered deleterious to health (see Chapter 6).

Persons who become physically less active need to reduce their energy intake to maintain ideal body weight, which in many cases may necessitate a reduction in dietary fat. On the other hand, normal individuals in energy balance appear to be capable of consuming high fat diets without adverse effects.

The physiology of fat digestion and absorption has been elucidated in considerable detail in recent years. The degree of utilization by normal individuals of naturally occurring or processed food fats and oils is greater than 90% (the ability of infants and children to utilize fats is considered in Chapter 3). Being the most concentrated form of food energy, the fat content of a diet generally determines its energy density. Diets with a very low energy density may be too voluminous to permit consumption of an amount sufficient to meet energy requirements, particularly for children. Diets based on root crops, plantains or cereals (especially when the germ has been removed) may fall into this category. Increasing the energy density of such diets by the addition of fat should be beneficial (see Chapter 3); the same objective could be achieved by increasing the availability and consumption of those foods which are naturally good sources of fat and other nutrients.

Fat as an energy source for work

It is well established that muscle does not utilize significant amounts of protein and that glucose from muscle glycogen and free fatty acids transported from adipose stores serve as the primary fuels for work. Adipose fat is the principal energy store of the body, and so most of the energy at low levels of exercise is derived from the transport of free fatty acids. With light or moderate exercise, of an intermittent nature, the proportion of fat and carbohydrate in the diet has no effect on performance (5).

Carbohydrate is almost exclusively oxidized in sustained activity near the maximum workload (as in some athletic competitions where the workload demands more than 80% of maximum oxygen uptake). Glycogen stores are sufficient only for about one to two hours of maximum workload. When the available muscle glycogen stores are utilized, efficiency falls rapidly and hypoglycaemia occurs. Concomitantly, the respiratory quotient declines and the muscle progressively depends on the free fatty acids for its energy (5). Under such extreme conditions, high-carbohydrate/low-fat diets are desirable to maintain blood sugar levels. At lower work levels (below 80% of maximum oxygen uptake) a more balanced intake of carbohydrate and fat is satisfactory, and sustained activity can be performed without difficulty, as both fatty acids and glucose are utilized.

Much information on the physiology of work has been obtained with subjects participating in athletic competitions or under training and frequently consuming a high-protein diet. These results must be applied with caution to conditions of manual labour. Few studies have been made on the relation between dietary intake and workload under free-living conditions. Finnish lumbermen selected a slightly higher percentage of energy as fat than workers in the camp who were engaged in lighter activities (6); however, military personnel on manoeuvres in the Canadian Arctic did not select a higher proportion of fat than troops with lower levels of physical activity in a temperate climate (7). Fat provided about 40% of energy in both studies. It thus appears that under a variety of types of manual labour classified as "heavy," diets relatively high in fat permit satisfactory performance, assuming of course that the "heavy" manual work does not in practice approach the type of sustained activity near maximum workload referred to earlier. There seems to be little evidence of any effect of the source of dietary energy on industrial work performance, provided that total energy needs are met.

Geographic factors and dietary fat

Observations in the past on groups subsisting in very cold climates probably gave rise to notions that such environments lead to a desire or need for higher fat intakes than warm or temperate climates (7). The high fat intake of such groups, however, was inherent in the available food, primarily of animal origin, which was high in protein and fat and low in carbohydrate. Conversely, most of the populations living in hot climates of the world subsist on low fat diets, again dictated by the available food sources. A series of studies with United States and Canadian army food rations at locations throughout the world showed a constant proportion of protein, fat and carbohydrate (9). This indicates that neither temperature nor humidity influenced the proportion of these nutrients. There thus appears to be no substantial evidence that climatic factors, temperature in particular, lead to changes in preference for the amount of dietary fat.

High-fat diets in weight reduction

Diets of high fat content (ketogenic diets) have been advocated for weight reduction in obese individuals. There is, however, no proof that

12

high-fat diets lead to greater loss of body fat than isocaloric diets containing usual proportions of fat, carbohydrates and proteins. Moreover, the use of high-fat diets has undesirable effects on blood lipid levels and should be discouraged (10).

Desirable levels of dietary fat

The wide range of dietary fat consumed throughout the world has been mentioned above. In the developing countries, there is evidence that in the lowest income groups, with dietary fat comprising about 10% of the energy, an increase to 15 to 20 energy % of fat, with adequate regard for essential fatty acids, would have beneficial effects. The importance of this conclusion in child and maternal nutrition is discussed in Chapters 3 and 5. In the developed countries, although many physically active individuals appear to tolerate diets containing more than 40% of the dietary energy as fat with no apparent health problems, sizeable fractions of the population are afflicted with several degenerative diseases in which the amount and types of dietary fat are implicated (see Chapter 6). In these populations there is substantial evidence that positive health benefits would be achieved by decreasing dietary fat to 30–35% of calories and by increasing the ratio of polyunsaturated to saturated fatty acids of the diet to 1:1.

3. THE USE OF FAT IN ADULT AND CHILD FEEDING

Pregnancy and fat intake

During pregnancy there are increased requirements of energy, protein and other nutrients for growth and for a maternal energy store in the form of fat, which is subsequently used in lactation. The additional needs for energy gradually increase from 150 kcal (0.63 MJ) per day in the first trimester to 350 kcal (1.5 MJ) per day in the second and third trimesters, with an average of 285 kcal (1.2 MJ) per day over the total 280 days. It is estimated that the total additional energy requirements are 80 000 kcal (335 MJ) for the whole period of pregnancy (11).

Data from some developing countries have indicated that average energy intakes in many pregnant women range from 60% to 80% of the recommended allowances (*see* 12–16). Among the causes of these inadequate energy intakes are poverty, cultural practices and beliefs and low energy density foods. In these countries the mean birth weight of offspring born to undernourished mothers is approximately 2.7 kg compared with an average of over 3 kg for those born to well-nourished mothers (*see* 17–21). The dietary energy derived from fat by mothers in many developing countries does not exceed 15%. It is known that additional energy is required during the first trimester, at which time there may be a reduced food intake. Consideration should therefore be given to increasing the energy density of the diets throughout pregnancy. (The role of essential fatty acids is discussed in Chapter 5.)

Lactation and fat intake

Breast milk has an energy content of approximately 0.70 kcal (2.9 kJ)/ml, and the average daily production from well-nourished lactating women is approximately 850 ml (ranging up to 1 000 ml). As the efficiency of the mammary gland to produce milk is about 80%, an additional energy intake ranging from 745 to 875 kcal (3.1–3.7 MJ) per day is recommended (11) to cover the energy cost of lactation. During a six-month period, the total energy required for milk production will be from 134 000–157 000 kcal (560–657 MJ). As a 36 000 kcal (151 MJ) reserve of body fat accumulates during pregnancy, an additional 100 000–120 000 kcal (418–502

MJ) will be required during a 180 day lactation period, or 550–660 kcal (2.3–2.8 MJ) per day.

Maternal nutrition during lactation can influence the amount and quality of milk available to the infant. The fatty acid composition of milk from mothers consuming a low-fat/high-carbohydrate diet may have a lower content of essential fatty acids, although the total fat content remains constant, provided that energy requirements are met. In extreme malnutrition, as observed in some East African mothers (22), total fat content may fall to about one half the normal, or even lower; in such cases, increased energy density of food is required.

The problems of protein-calorie malnutrition

Protein-calorie malnutrition (PCM) is of concern to public health authorities in many developing countries (23–25). It is particularly widespread among older infants and young children. When breast-feeding is not practised, inadequate formula feeding may precipitate protein-calorie malnutrition in the first few months of life. It has been estimated that several tens of million children of preschool age suffer from this condition to varying degrees.[1] Mortality is high, and in the chronic, mild and moderate forms, morphological and functional changes occur, which, depending upon the age of onset and duration, can have irreversible consequences in later life. Energy malnutrition in adult women of child-bearing age can affect not only pregnancy outcome and foetal development but also lactation performance (26–29). In adults of both sexes engaged in moderate to heavy physical labour, inadequate energy intake limits energy expenditure in everyday activities (30).

The underlying causes of malnutrition are poverty, inadequate food availability and general social underdevelopment, which lead to consumption of diets inadequate in both quality and quantity. The nutrition problem is aggravated by the sociological setting and by frequent episodes of repeated infections that act synergistically with malnutrition. Undernutrition is aggravated by infections that by themselves are responsible for a large proportion of deaths during infancy and childhood.

Until a decade ago it was widely believed that childhood malnutrition was due primarily to insufficiency of protein in the diet. There is now adequate evidence to show that the most limiting factor is *not* protein but *energy*. In a sizeable proportion of children, however, both energy and protein are inadequate because of the very small amounts of food consumed; but in these same children the extent of *energy deficit is greater than that of protein*. This finding has practical implications in the control and prevention of the problem (31–33).

---

[1] United Nations World Food Conference, Rome, November 1974, E/CONF 65/3.

Fat intake in infants

INFANTS BREAST-FED BY WELL-NOURISHED MOTHERS

In well-nourished mothers breast milk alone satisfies the nutritional needs of normal human infants up to the age of about five months. After this it is necessary to introduce supplementary foods, but breast milk should continue as an important source of food until production ceases. Breast milk, because of its balanced amino acid composition, complements vegetable (cereals and pulses) proteins, thus increasing their net protein utilization. Moreover, it provides ideal hygienic conditions for infant nutrition and health; unlike cow's milk, it has the appropriate composition for the human infant. For example, human milk has a higher content of fat and EFA and a lower content of protein and minerals than cow's milk. Specific proteins and fats in human milk promote the absorption of calcium and iron, and milk lipase facilitates the digestion of fats. Human milk also offers protection against infection through the secretion of antibodies, and the bifidus factor. Furthermore, the environmental conditions in the intestine favour the development of lactobacillus rather than *E. coli*, thus protecting against invasion by pathogenic strains of *E. coli* and gastroenteritis (33a).

In well-nourished mothers the fat in breast milk contributes 50–60% and protein about 6–7% of the total energy intake of their infants. The proportion of protein to the total energy content ensures optimum protein utilization (13).

Considering the mean protein and energy content of breast milk of optimum composition on the one hand and the recommended energy intake and safe levels of protein intakes in infants (11) on the other, an intake of 1 000 ml of milk per day would cease to satisfy the recommended intakes at about four months of age. In view of the fact that growth rates of healthy infants who are solely breast-fed are satisfactory up to the age of five or six months, the current recommended allowances appear to be somewhat high, particularly when it is realized that daily milk production is most often less than 1 000 ml and closer to 850 ml in well-nourished mothers.

FAILURE IN LACTATION

Under conditions of inadequate breast milk secretion, the early introduction of supplementary feeding to infants assumes paramount importance. The questions arise as to what the supplementary intake should be in terms of nutrients and through which foods this can be achieved. There are two alternatives: (*i*) bottle-feeding of milk and/or formulated

16

foods, and (ii) administration of locally available food mixes prepared as thin gruels that can be spoon-fed. Whichever system is chosen, an energy content of around 50–60 kcal (0.21–0.25 MJ)/g of protein should be aimed at.

The addition of fat is essential under either alternative. As far as is known, there are no data on the maximum amount of fat that small infants can tolerate; but small, severely malnourished children tolerate up to 70% of energy as fat, even in the presence of partially impaired fat absorption. Two-month-old infants are able to absorb 50–60 energy % of fat from human milk with an efficiency greater than 85%; similar absorption figures are obtained from vegetable oils, such as maize oil. Based on these considerations, home-made preparations as supplementary foods are being studied (see Appendix 2). Careful consideration should be given to the type of fat (e.g., essential fatty acid and vitamin E-adequate fats) and to the possible risk of force feeding, directly or indirectly, in order to satisfy water needs. These risks include obesity and diminished desire of the infant to suck the breast.

The failure of mothers to breast-feed their infants in early life poses a very special and serious problem in developing countries. In families migrating to urban areas the practice of breast-feeding tends to decline, mainly because of socio-economic pressures and a desire toward "modernization." Consequently, formula milks are resorted to, with the inherent danger of infection from contaminated bottles and overdilution of feeds for reasons of economy.

Unfortunately, foods available in most homes in developing countries cannot supply the nutrients obtained by the infant from breast milk, as diets based on cereals and legumes are too bulky to meet the protein and energy needs of infants under four months of age. The early introduction of infant formulas in the form of home-made supplementary foods (see Appendix 2) therefore becomes very important.

It is concluded that the development of "weaning food" mixtures in developing countries can be useful under such conditions. Special care must be taken to provide enough energy to the child by increasing the energy density of such formulas. Addition of vegetable fats adequate in essential fatty acids and vitamin E can overcome the relative energy deficit of such diets. Total energy per gram of protein in the fat-enriched mixtures should ideally provide between 50 and 60 kcal (0.21–0.25 MJ)/g of protein.

Fat absorption in infancy

In normal children, particularly during the first month of life, there are difficulties in the digestion and absorption of certain fats. Such absorption depends on (a) the chemical properties of the fat and (b) the digestive and absorptive characteristics of the individual, which normally depend on age.

Absorption of fat in children can be summarized as follows:

(a) *Factors dependent on the nature of fat*

(i) Vegetable fats containing polyunsaturated fatty acids are better absorbed than saturated fats.

(ii) Fats containing medium-chain (8–12 carbon chain length) and short-chain (less than 8 carbon chain length) fatty acids are more easily absorbed than those containing longer chains.

(iii) The pancreatic lipase, which hydrolyses fatty acids preferentially in the 1 and 3 positions of the triglycerides, produces free fatty acids and 2-monoglycerides; the absorption of certain fatty acids in the 2 position is thereby favoured (34). This holds for palmitic acid, which in breast milk predominates in position 2, while in cow's milk it is uniformly distributed in positions 1, 2 and 3. This fact and the presence of lipase in human milk explain in part the better absorption of fat from human milk than from cow's milk (35).

(b) *Factors dependent on the individual*

(i) Pancreatic lipase activity can be detected in early gestation and increases progressively with age (36). However, feeds rich in protein in the neonatal period accelerate the development of pancreatic lipase; colostrum can play an important role in this process (37).

(ii) Bile acid concentration in the duodenal fluid of newborns is below 2 mmol per litre, which is the critical micellar concentration (38). Despite this fact, human milk is still well absorbed (39).

(iii) Moderate to severe protein-calorie deficiency states are accompanied by slight to moderate decreases in fat absorption. The significance of the subclinical malabsorption syndrome or tropical enteropathy, which appears to be widespread in children and adults of tropical countries, remains to be established (40). The fat absorption capacity of underweight newborn infants (small for date) in relation to premature and to normal infants also needs to be determined.

Fats in the feeding of young children

Diets of young children from poor families often do not provide enough energy and may also be deficient in protein. It is possible, though improbable, for such children to satisfy their needs of both energy and protein by merely increasing the quantity of the food they consume, without significantly changing the quality. Practical problems arise because the diets contain low amounts of fat and therefore have a low energy density. Consequently, children, particularly in the younger age group, often find it difficult to consume the large volumes of food necessary to satisfy their energy needs. This difficulty can be overcome by increasing the frequency of feeding (41). In many households this may not be possible because the mothers go out to work and cannot devote enough time and attention to supervising the frequent feeding of their children. Under these circumstances it is important to reduce the bulk of the diet by increasing the energy density. A rational way of doing this would be to increase the fat content of the diet. This situation changes in older children, who can eat larger volumes of food relative to their energy needs.

Severe malnutrition impairs a number of physiological functions, among these, intestinal absorption of nutrients, including dietary fat. It appears, however, that impaired fat absorption is not a critical factor in mildly and moderately undernourished children (41a).

When diets that provide 66% or more of the energy as fat are consumed by children beyond the rapid growth phase (about one year), ketosis occurs, which means that the upper limit of fat in a diet clearly has to be below this level (42). Furthermore, the inclusion of large amounts of fat would necessitate a reduction in the amounts of other food items that are sources of essential nutrients, such as vitamins and minerals. This is an important consideration in determining the maximum amount of fat as an energy source.

The energy-protein ratio of the diet is also an important criterion. The segment of child populations that consumes diets providing enough protein but inadequate energy will benefit from the addition of fat. But children whose intakes of both protein and energy are unsatisfactory would be at risk of *not* having their protein needs met if the energy gap were covered through fat alone — an undesirable situation. An appreciable proportion of children falls into this category; in several developing countries nearly one third of the undernourished child population belongs to this group (32, 43). Under these circumstances it would be desirable to provide part of the additional energy through fat and the rest by increasing the amount of the diet consumed so as to increase protein intakes as well. The amount of fat or fat-rich foods that should be added to provide the additionally needed energy must also take into account the EFA needs of children in this age group.

Diets of children in several developing countries provide between 10 and 15 energy % as fat, and the energy deficit in children consuming such diets varies from 20% to 30% of recommended allowances, depending upon age.

If the entire energy deficit were to be covered through added fats, the contribution of fats to total energy would rise to between 35% and 40% — a figure which appears high in the light of health risks in adults. If one half the energy shortfall were covered by additional amounts of added fat and the other half by an increase in the quantity of the diet being consumed, energy from fat would then account for about 25% of total dietary energy. In Central America maize-bean based diets fed *ad libitum* to children between the ages of 15 and 30 months fulfilled protein and energy needs when the diets contained 22% of total energy as fats (14% visible and 8% invisible). At this level it should also be possible to meet the EFA requirements (see Chapters 4 and 5).

An important practical consideration in promoting the use of fats in the diets of children, particularly in developing countries, is the availability and cost of edible fat. In many, but not all, the production of fat is limited and the per caput availability low. Furthermore, in some countries edible fat is an expensive food item and the level of fat consumption shows a marked dependence on income. The frequency distribution of fat intake is therefore highly skewed. Children whose diets do not provide adequate energy intakes belong to the poorest income groups, and these are the very children whose diets need to be made energy dense with fat — which they cannot afford.

Although it is desirable to improve the energy content and energy density of diets of young children by the inclusion of fat, this recommendation is unlikely to find immediate application in countries where large segments of the population live under economic constraints that do not permit them sufficient quantities of even the cheapest foods to fulfil their needs. This does not diminish the merits of the recommendation, but indicates that in developing countries there is an urgent need to increase the per caput availability of edible fats and energy-rich foods at a cost which permits equitable distribution.

4. ESSENTIAL FATTY ACIDS

Introduction

A dietary fat deficiency syndrome was first recognized and described in the classical papers by Burr and Burr (44, 45), who proposed that linoleic acid (18:2, n–6) and possibly α-linolenic acid (18:3, n–3) were essential fatty acids (EFA); however, in studies on EFA the main emphasis has been on linoleic acid (18:2, n–6). In recent years the discovery of the prostaglandins, thromboxanes and prostacyclin has given further insight into the physiological functions of EFA. Furthermore, recent studies have shown that α-linolenic acid (18:3, n–3) may have specific functions in certain tissues and therefore merits careful study.

Metabolism

Essential fatty acids are necessary for the normal functions of all tissues. They must be present in the diet because animals, including man, cannot introduce the n–3 and n–6 double bonds (see Chapter 1). Dietary linoleic (18:2, n–6) and α-linolenic (18:3, n–3) acids are metabolized by desaturation and chain elongation to long-chain EFA derivatives, resulting in two families of n–6 and n–3 acids, which are involved in the structures and functions of all tissues. In the absence of EFA, animals introduce double bonds in stearic acid (18:0), but only starting from the n–9 position. The result is oleic acid (18:1, n–9), which is subsequently further desaturated and chain elongated to an eicosatrienoic acid (20:3, n–9), producing a third family of polyunsaturated fatty acids. Simplified metabolic pathways for the three families of fatty acids are illustrated in Figure 2.

It should be noted that dihomo-γ-linolenic (20:3, n–6), arachidonic (20:4, n–6) and eicosapentaenoic (20:5, n–3) acids can be converted into the prostaglandin families. The 20 and 22 carbon fatty acids of n–6 and n–3 families are preferentially incorporated in the cell membrane phospholipids, where they have an important structural and functional role.

The presence of α-linolenic acid (18:3, n–3) inhibits the desaturation of linoleic acid (18:2, n–6) and that of oleic acid (18:1, n–9) to a greater extent; similarly, linoleic acid (18:2, n–6) inhibits the desaturation of

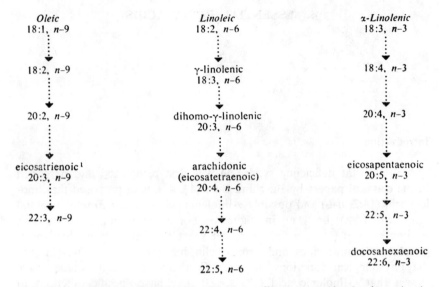

Oleic 18:1, *n*–9	Linoleic 18:2, *n*–6	α-Linolenic 18:3, *n*–3
18:2, *n*–9	γ-linolenic 18:3, *n*–6	18:4, *n*–3
20:2, *n*–9	dihomo-γ-linolenic 20:3, *n*–6	20:4, *n*–3
eicosatrienoic[1] 20:3, *n*–9	arachidonic (eicosatetraenoic) 20:4, *n*–6	eicosapentaenoic 20:5, *n*–3
22:3, *n*–9	22:4, *n*–6	22:5, *n*–3
	22:5, *n*–6	docosahexaenoic 22:6, *n*–3

[1] Normally, negligible amounts of oleic acid (18:1, *n*–9) are converted to its eicosatrienoic (20:3, *n*–9) derivative, but significant conversion does occur when there is an EFA deficiency in the diet. The ratio of this eicosatrienoic acid (20:3, *n*–9) to arachidonic acid (eicosatetraenoic acid, 20:4, *n*–6) can then be used as an index of the deficiency; this ratio is referred to as the triene/tetraene ratio (see also page 28).

FIGURE 2. Simplified metabolic pathways.

oleic acid (18:1, *n*–9). Therefore, in diets containing both linoleic (18:2, *n*–6) and α-linolenic acids (18:3, *n*–3), only negligible conversion of oleic (18:1, *n*–9) to eicosatrienoic acid (20:3, *n*–9) can occur.

Conversion factor for long-chain essential fatty acids

Studies *in vivo* have shown that the Δ6 desaturation of linoleic acid (18:2, *n*–6) is the rate-limiting step in the synthesis of arachidonic acid (78). The efficiency of desaturation is different in different species. The rat has a highly efficient desaturation mechanism, but linoleic acid (18:2, *n*–6) has no EFA activity for the cat, which has an obligatory requirement for the longer-chain polyunsaturated fatty acids (79).

There is evidence that the rate limitations in desaturations observed in animals are also found in man (80). Because man is genetically polymorphic it is to be expected that different efficiencies of conversion will be found between individuals and according to the disease status.

Fatty acids are utilized in the body as a principal source of energy.

Hence a proportion of dietary essential fatty acids is also oxidized for energy. Furthermore, dietary linoleic (18:2, n–6) and α-linolenic (18:3, n–3) acids have been shown to be distributed after ingestion between adipose fat triglycerides, other tissue stores and tissue structural lipid. By contrast, the long-chain essential fatty acids, arachidonic (20:4, n–6) and docosahexaenoic (22:6, n–3), are preferentially incorporated into the structural lipid and are spared from oxidation (81).

Dietary arachidonic (20:4, n–6) and docosahexaenoic (22:6, n–3) acids are incorporated into structural lipids about 20 times more efficiently than they are incorporated after synthesis from dietary linoleic (18:2, n–6) and α-linolenic (18:3, n–3) acids (82, 83). Because of these overall limitations in the metabolism of the parent acids of 18 carbon chain length to their long-chain derivatives, a conversion factor should be considered.

Essential fatty acid deficiency syndrome

The most complete description of EFA deficiency symptoms has been obtained from studies in young rats (Table 2). Some of these symptoms have also been observed in EFA-deficient humans, such as abnormal skin conditions, reduced regeneration of tissues, increased susceptibility to infections and an increase in the triene/tetraene ratio [eicosatrienoic (20:3, n–9)/arachidonic (20:4, n–6) acids].

Essential fatty acid deficiency in humans

The classical studies by Hansen et al. (46–48) on EFA deficiency in infants and children with various skin disorders showed a curative effect on intractable eczema in many patients when the diet was supplemented with lard, maize oil or linseed oil. Although EFAs have not proved to be a general cure for eczema, these experiments indicated that they might be a necessary nutrient in human diets. In a later study (49) with healthy infants, formula diets varying in linoleic (18:2, n–6) acid content from less than 0.1 to 7.3 energy % were used. These studies showed that dermal changes were not observed when 1 energy % or more was fed as linoleic acid (18:2, n–6). On this basis it was concluded that the minimum requirement for EFAs in humans was 1 energy % or more to cure the skin symptoms. In recent years, intravenous alimentation using glucose and amino acid mixtures has been shown to induce EFA deficiency in humans (50, 52). Furthermore, EFAs are probably necessary for the healing of surgical wounds (e.g., in intestinal resections), in the healing of entero-cutaneous fistulae and in severe burn cases (53, 54).

α-Linolenic acid as an essential fatty acid

Although a specific deficiency of α-linolenic acid (18:3, *n*–3) has not been observed in humans or rats, experimental evidence with laboratory rats indicates that this fatty acid and especially the 20 and 22 carbon chain length acids (long-chain fatty acids) derived from it have a specific role in the development and function of the brain (55) and retina (56). Dietary α-linolenic acid (18:3, *n*–3) has been shown to prevent skin lesion in monkeys even in the presence of dietary linoleic acid (18:2, *n*–6; see reference 57), and is the EFA in rainbow trout in which linoleic acid has no beneficial effect (57a).

Because of the possible specific role of this family of fatty acids in the specialized tissues, α-linolenic acid (18:3, *n*–3) should be considered an essential dietary constituent. However, more research is needed in clarifying the role of the α-linolenic acid family in human nutrition.

Essential fatty acid requirement

Linoleic (18:2, *n*–6) and α-linolenic (18:3, *n*–3) acids differ with respect to their biological activities (see Table 2). Furthermore, the validity of extrapolation to the human infant from data obtained with newly weaned, rapidly growing rats is open to question, and even more so extrapolation to the adult human. For the human infant a dietary intake of at least 3 energy % of linoleic acid can be considered adequate (see Chapter 5); however, this level is significantly lower than the average linoleic acid (18:2, *n*–6) concentration in human milk. The efficiency of α-linolenic acid (18:3, *n*–3) with respect to growth is somewhat less than that of linoleic acid; on the other hand, the derivatives of linoleic acid [γ-linolenic acid (18:3, *n*–6); dihomo-γ-linolenic acid (20:3, *n*–6) and arachidonic acid (20:4, *n*–6)] are more effective (58, 58a, 58b).

For human adults a dietary intake of at least 3 energy % as EFA is recommended. However, many factors are known to increase EFA requirements (see below). Moreover, in populations having a high incidence of atherosclerosis (see Chapter 6), much higher amounts of EFA may be required.

Interactions between essential fatty acids and other dietary constituents

Because EFAS never occur alone in fats or foods, it is necessary to consider possible interactions between them and other nutrients which may affect the requirement or utilization of them. Most investigations of interactions have been made on laboratory animals, but the phenomena observed are considered to operate also in humans (59).

TABLE 2. – ESSENTIAL FATTY ACID DEFICIENCY SYMPTOMS

Symptoms	Efficiency ratio linoleic (18:2, n–6)/ α-linolenic (18:3, n–3) [1]
Reduced growth rate	1
Abnormal skin conditions: scaliness (parakeratosis) dermatitis increased water loss	about 10
Sterility in males and females	?
Kidney abnormalities: papillary necrosis and haematuria renal hypertension	?
Mitochondria: abnormal swelling of mitochondria abnormal mitochondrial function causing decreased food efficiency	about 3
Decreased capillary resistance and increased fragility of erythrocytes	1
Increased water consumption	about 10
Biochemical abnormalities: increase in triene/tetraene ratio above 0.1 decreased prostaglandin biosynthesis resulting in a significant reduction in physiological functions of tissue, such as the heart, platelets, adipose tissue	100
Increased susceptibility to infection	?

[1] The effectiveness of linoleic (18:2, n–6) and α-linolenic (18:3, n–3) acids in reversing individual signs of EFA deficiency has been expressed as a ratio where the data exist.

1. *Dietary saturated fatty acids* have been observed to increase the requirement of EFAS as measured by growth, dermal symptoms of deficiency and the triene/tetraene ratio in tissue lipids. The magnitude of the effect is small because relatively large changes in content of saturated fatty acids are necessary to induce small changes in these indicators of EFA deficiency. Increasing saturated fatty acids in the diet of man increases the level of serum cholesterol (60) and the thrombotic activity of blood platelets, which can be counteracted by linoleic acid (61).

2. *Cis-monounsaturated acids* partially replace EFAS in the lipids of EFA-deficient animals and humans. They likewise suppress the utilization

25

of EFAs when they are present at high dietary levels. For example, the principal one, oleic acid (18:1, n–9), when present at 10 times the amount of linoleic acid (18:2, n–6), induces a triene/tetraene ratio of 1, which indicates a clear EFA deficiency (68).

3. *Isomeric unsaturated fatty acids*, such as positional isomers of oleic acid (18:1, n–9), occur in small amounts in partially hydrogenated edible oils. This series of cis 18:1 isomers and an isomeric series of cis, cis-methylene interrupted linoleic acid (18:2, n–6) isomers have been tested as substrates in several enzyme and biological systems. Each system tested displays a unique pattern of specificity or utilization. For a given system, some isomers are good substrates and others are not. Each isomer is recognized by a different biological system. The position of a double bond governs the metabolism of a fatty acid.

Trans isomers of unsaturated fatty acids are produced during partial hydrogenation of oils and are present in ruminant fats. A range of positional isomers is found in these products. The trans isomers are known to be well utilized for energy. They occur in structural lipids of animals and humans consuming partially hydrogenated oils without consequences. The trans acids occur predominantly in the 1 position of tissue phospholipids in the place of saturated acids. Their metabolic pathways are somewhat different from their corresponding cis isomers. Trans-monounsaturated acids have been found to increase the EFA requirement in animals when included at moderate levels in the diet (62).

4. *Polyunsaturated acids* belong to several families, each arising from a different precursor (Fig. 2). Linoleic acid (18:2, n–6) yields a family of acids which all have the n–6 structure, and α-linolenic acid (18:3, n–3) yields a family with n–3 structure. In the absence of these two families in the diet, a family of n–9 acids derived from oleic acid (18:1, n–9) occurs in abnormally high amounts. There is no metabolic crossover from one family to another. Low concentrations of α-linolenic acid (18:3, n–3) are very effective in suppressing the metabolism of linoleic acid (18:2, n–6). Moderate levels of linoleic acid (18:2, n–6) inhibit the metabolism of α-linolenic acid (18:3, n–3). Oleic acid (18:1, n–9) suppresses the metabolism of linoleic acid (18:2, n–6) only at high levels of the former. The competitive properties of these families are: α-linolenic (18:3, n–3) >linoleic (18:2, n–6) >oleic (18:1, n–9) acids. These interactions were observed in studies using pure fatty acids and have been confirmed under conditions in which all common fatty acids are present in the diet. These studies

indicated that each type of dietary fatty acid influences the utilization of the others. The composition of dietary fat controls the metabolism of polyunsaturated fatty acids and therefore the metabolic activities of the intracellular membranes containing them.

5. *Cholesterol* is not a required nutrient. An increased serum cholesterol level has been found to accentuate EFA deficiency, probably because it may deplete the EFA pool available for phospholipids. Dietary EFAS are also effective in reducing serum cholesterol levels.

6. *Protein* is required for synthesis of lipoproteins of serum and cellular membranes. Inadequate intakes of protein may reduce growth and delay onset of overt symptoms of EFA deficiency and may contribute to faulty lipid transport. Protein nutrition and metabolism must be normal for EFA metabolism to be normal, because lipoproteins are involved in EFA metabolism and transport.

7. *Carbohydrates*, according to studies of EFA deficiency, may replace EFAS in the diet. The nature of the carbohydrate component of the diet has been found to have little influence upon the development of the deficiency; the signs are traceable to the lack of EFAS rather than to the abundance of sucrose. EFA deficiency was induced in humans by long-term intravenous feeding with fat-free preparations containing glucose, whereas preparations free of glucose did not induce a deficiency. The constant infusion of glucose without EFAS inhibits their release from adipose tissue due to increased insulin levels, so that the reserve of EFAS is unavailable. Under these conditions, an EFA deficiency can be detected within a week.

The abnormal metabolism of lipids and carbohydrates in diabetics also involves EFAS. Experimental diabetes accelerates EFA deficiency, and fatty acid patterns of serum lipids of diabetics are modified in the direction of EFA deficiency.

8. *Vitamin E* protects the EFAS in body tissues against peroxidative loss. Since increased intakes of EFAS generally increase the tissue content of polyunsaturated fatty acids, there will be an increased need for vitamin E, as has been observed in the premature infant (63). Animal experiments indicate that dietary vegetable fats contain adequate amounts of vitamin E to meet the increased tissue need for this vitamin when such fats are fed. Vitamin E also stabilizes vegetable fats against rancidity during processing and storage and thus prevents the loss of EFAS in those fats.

Possible adverse effects of polyunsaturated fats

There has been concern that a relatively high intake of dietary fat, especially of polyunsaturated fats, may be an environmental factor in some human cancers. Animal experiments have shown that, when fed with a carcinogen, polyunsaturated fats are more co-carcinogenic than saturated fats (64). The addition of synthetic antioxidants could significantly reduce the co-carcinogenicity (65).

The evidence from several human studies does not support a relationship between cancer incidence and type of dietary fat (66). Epidemiological data have attempted to correlate the incidence of certain human gastrointestinal cancers and the intake of dietary fat, but the correlations are not entirely consistent. These observations, together with the animal experiments, have stimulated considerable current research to clarify the possible role of dietary fat in human carcinogenesis.

A possible increased predisposition to gallstone formation has been reported in men who consumed a low-cholesterol, high-polyunsaturated fat diet for several years (67). Laboratory animal experiments have produced the opposite results. Further evaluation of this possible relationship in humans should be made.

Assessment of essential fatty acid status in humans

The severe clinical manifestations of EFA deficiency in humans, which have been reviewed in detail (59, 68), include eczematous lesions, refractive impetigo, dry scaly skin, coarse and sparse hair, frequent stools, perianal irritation, oozing in the intertriginous folds, and generalized erythema. These symptoms are variable and are not useful for quantified estimates of EFA status or intake.

Several biochemical measures of EFA status have been developed for animals (59, 69) and extended to humans (59, 68). The ratio of triene/tetraene in serum lipids has been used as an indicator of EFA status in humans (70), but the method of analysis then used is now obsolete. Currently, the ratio of the eicosatrienoic acid (20:3, n–9) to arachidonic acid (20:4, n–6) of serum phospholipids measured by gas liquid chromatography is preferred (68).[1] The average ratio measured on a population of 236 Americans, hospitalized for nonmetabolic causes, was found to be approximately 0.1 ± 0.08; none of the individuals had a ratio as high

---

[1] To measure the triene/tetraene ratio, it might be preferable to use the phosphatidyl choline fraction of serum lipids instead of total phospholipids. If packed columns are used for the gas liquid chromatography, then saturated or monounsaturated fatty acids from serum sphingomyelin may co-chromatograph with the triene, giving a higher apparent value.

28

as 0.4, the limit of normality set in 1964 using a less precise method. Only minor differences were found between males and females. For the population studied, the upper limit of normality must therefore be set at least as low as 0.2, the average plus the standard deviation. This value may be higher than is found in adequate EFA status, for there is no guarantee that the population from which it was derived is truly normal. The value can be used for comparisons between individuals and populations, but cannot be used to decide normality. The lower the triene/tetraene ratio, the better the EFA status.

Several other parameters based upon analysis of fatty acids of serum lipids are useful for assessing EFA status. Individual fatty acids vary in concentration in serum lipids in response to level of dietary EFA. In EFA deficiency, palmitoleic acid (16:1, n–7), oleic acid (18:1, n–9) and eicosatrienoic acid (20:3, n–9) are significantly increased, while linoleic acid (18:2, n–6), dihomo-γ-linolenic acid (20:3, n–6) and arachidonic acid (20:4, n–6) are significantly decreased.

In EFA deficiency, minor changes are noted in other fatty acids, but parameters even more useful for assessment of status may be calculated from the fatty acid patterns. Thus there is a marked decrease (68, 71) in (a) the double bond index (number of double bonds per fatty acid molecule), (b) the total n–6 acids, and (c) the sum of linoleic acid (18:2, n–6) plus arachidonic acid (20:4, n–6) minus eicosatrienoic acid (20:3, n–9). The linoleic acid (18:2, n–6) content of serum cholesteryl esters has also been used as a measure of EFA status (72, 73).

The recent dietary intake of linoleic acid (18:2, n–6) of an individual may be estimated by the equation

$$\log_{10} \text{linoleic acid} = 0.079 \, [18{:}2 \, (n{-}6) + 20{:}4 \, (n{-}6) - 20{:}3 \, (n{-}9)] - 1.9$$

in which linoleic acid (18:2, n–6) is expressed as energy % and the other three fatty acids are expressed as % of fatty acids in serum phospholipids of infants. Using this equation, the intake of linoleic acid (18:2, n–6) of normal breast-fed infants was estimated to be 5.1 energy %.

The total n–6 acids of serum phospholipids are also useful for estimating linoleic acid (18:2, n–6) intake according to the following equation:

$$\log_{10} \text{linoleic acid} = 5.8 \, (\log_{10} \text{total } n{-}6) - 8.5.$$

With this equation the intake of linoleic acid (18:2, n–6) of normal breast-fed infants was estimated to be 4.8 energy %. The values of apparent dietary intake of linoleic acid, calculated by either of these equations, may be compared with the recommended allowance (see Chapter 5) to assess the EFA status of an individual.

5. THE ROLE OF ESSENTIAL FATTY ACIDS IN EARLY DEVELOPMENT

The structural lipids

Dietary fat is important in foetal and early infant growth because this is the period of organogenesis, when there is a high essential fatty acid demand for the synthesis of cell structural lipid. This is true especially for the central nervous system, in which the main period of cell division is prenatal.

The two most important structural components of all cell structures are protein and lipid. Because both linoleic (18:2, *n*–6) and α-linolenic (18:3, *n*–3) acids and their long-chain derivatives are found in foetal and neonate structural lipids in the human (in the ratio of *n*–6 to *n*–3 acids ranging between 5 and 7 to 1), both families of fatty acids should be provided in the diet.

Considerations in pregnancy

There are no studies on human essential fatty acid requirements in pregnancy and lactation. The additional demand for uterine, placental and foetal growth, together with the increased maternal blood volume and mammary gland development, will have to be met from the maternal diet. On the foetal side of the placenta the blood phospholipids have a higher content of long-chain fatty acids (74, 75). The fat in the foetal organs, especially the liver and brain, is structural and contains a high proportion of phospholipid; the essential fatty acids in these phospholipids are mainly long-chain (75, 75a).

The approximate accumulation of essential fatty acids during pregnancy is about 623 g (Table 3), which is equivalent to an additional 0.95 energy % as essential fatty acids per day above the basic energy requirement of 2 200 kcal (9.2 MJ).

Requirement in pregnancy

The accumulation of the long-chain essential fatty acids in the foetus is achieved by a progressive increase in chain length and degree of

TABLE 3. – APPROXIMATE FAT AND ESSENTIAL FATTY ACID
GAIN IN GRAMS IN PREGNANCY AND FULL-TERM FOETUS
(3 500 g)

	Total fat	Essential fatty acid content
Maternal fat deposited	4 464	553
Foetus, placenta and increase in uterus, mammary gland and maternal blood:		
phospholipids	63	20
adipose fat	420	50
Total net gain in essential fatty acids		623 g

NOTE: The table has been derived from data in references 13, 76, 76a–d. The maternal fat gained during pregnancy contributes to milk production in the first hundred days of lactation (13). The essential fatty acid content of breast milk has therefore been used to calculate the appropriate proportions in the maternal fat stores — that is, 12.4% as total essential fatty acids (Table 4), which is in agreement with a small number of maternal adipose tissue analyses (76a).

unsaturation of essential fatty acids in maternal liver, placenta, foetal liver and foetal brain, resulting in high concentrations of arachidonic (20:4, n–6) and docosahexaenoic (22:6, n–3) acids in foetal tissues (75).

Maternal fat is accumulated primarily during the first and second trimesters as an energy and essential fatty acid reserve for lactation; foetal growth occurs mainly in the last two months of pregnancy. In Table 3 the total essential fatty acid gain in the mother and the foetus has been averaged over the whole pregnancy; however, because of the overall limitations discussed above and on page 22, it is suggested that the essential fatty acid intake recommended in pregnancy amounts approximately to an additional 1.5 energy % above the basic requirement for essential fatty acids.

Maternal malnutrition and prematurity

Several neurological and mental handicaps are associated with low birth weight at term. The highest incidence of low birth weight is found in lower socio-economic groups, which are often malnourished. In addition to the known effects of protein deprivation on foetal brain growth, experimental essential fatty acid deficiency has also been shown in rats to retard brain growth, alter brain function and increase perinatal mortality (84, 85, 86).

During growth there is an intimate link between protein and essential fatty acid deposition. Hence, the role of essential fatty acids and energy in the aetiology of low birth weight and the associated handicaps should be given serious consideration.

The premature infant, because of its rapid rate of growth and body fat deposition, particularly risks nutritional deficiency. Care should be taken to fulfil its requirements.

Considerations in lactation and infant feeding

A guide to "optimum" recommended intakes can be obtained from studies on human milk composition for consideration of requirements both for lactating mothers and for infants. The early data on the fatty acids in human milk suggested a wide variability in its composition, and owing to technical difficulties, few researchers analysed the long-chain essential fatty acids. In addition, the problems of sampling breast milk were not necessarily appreciated in terms of changes in composition during a single feeding and throughout lactation (22).

Data available on the milk fatty acid composition from five countries (Table 4; see also references 22, 77) and from five centres in the United Kingdom (77a) exhibit a remarkable degree of agreement. About 4–5% of the total energy is present as linoleic (18:2, n–6) and α-linolenic (18:3, n–3) acids (77a) and 1% as long-chain essential fatty acid derivatives, thus amounting to about 6% for all the essential fatty acids (22).

Requirement in lactation

During a six- to nine-month period of lactation a decline in the long-chain essential fatty acids of milk to less than 0.7 energy % has been observed (77); however, the milk output increases, so that approximately the same amount of long-chain essential fatty acids and more linoleic (18:2, n–6) and α-linolenic (18:3, n–3) acids may be secreted. The fat stored during normal pregnancy is utilized during lactation at the rate of approximately 200–300 kcal (0.84–1.3 MJ) per day over the first hundred days of lactation. If maternal food intake matches the recommended allowances for lactation, it can be assumed that most of the excess depot fat will be utilized for milk production. This means that during the first hundred days of lactation the increased dietary requirements for essential fatty acids would be two thirds the amount of essential fatty acids needed to replace total output in the milk.

As the efficiency of incorporation of dietary fatty acids into milk is unknown, the precise quantities replacing that which is secreted in the milk cannot be calculated. The actual replacement amount must be greater, however, than the total amount secreted. Based on the data on human milk composition, the amounts of the fatty acids to be replaced have been calculated in grams per day in Table 5.

Between 3 and 5 g of all essential fatty acids are secreted in the milk per day, part of this amount as long-chain essential fatty acids. To express the data in energy terms as parent essential fatty acids (linoleic 18:2, n-6 and α-linolenic 18:3, n-3 acids), the loss during their conversion to

TABLE 4. – COMPOSITION OF HUMAN MILK FATTY ACIDS [1]
(Results expressed as % of weight)

Fatty acid	Mean of the average for each country	Weighted mean	Standard error of the mean
10:0	2.5	2.5	± 0.3
12:0	8.0	6.8	± 0.7
14:0	11.0	11.0	± 1.1
16:0	25.0	25.0	± 0.6
16:1	2.0	1.9	± 0.2
18:0	6.2	6.4	± 0.3
18:1	30.0	32.0	± 1.1
18:2, n-6	9.2	9.1	± 0.5
18:3, n-3	0.9	0.8	± 0.1
Long-chain essential fatty acids:			
n-6 (20:3, n-6 + 20:4, n-6 + 22:4, n-6 + 22:5, n-6)	0.98	1.0	± 0.3
n-3 (20:5, n-3 + 22:5, n-3 + 22:6, n-3)	1.3	1.4	± 0.1

[1] Total number of samples 261, including 116 from the UK, 22 from Denmark, 18 from Sri Lanka, 67 from Tanzania and 38 from Uganda. Sampled between 4 and 6 weeks postpartum. Later the long-chain EFA decreases; however, more data are needed on the composition of milk at later periods.

34

TABLE 5. – ESSENTIAL FATTY ACIDS (EFA) IN HUMAN MILK
AT TWO DIFFERENT ENERGY LEVELS

Fatty acid	Energy as total EFA in milk	Grams/day in milk of	
		600 kcal (2.5 MJ)	810 kcal (3.4 MJ) [1]
Linoleic acid (18:2, *n*–6)	6	3.0	4.0
	4	2.0	2.7
α-Linolenic (18:3, *n*–3)	6	0.26	0.35
	4	0.18	0.23
Long-chain [2] EFA *n*–6	6	0.19	0.25
	4	0.16	0.21
Long-chain [2] EFA *n*–3	6	0.28	0.38
	4	0.19	0.25

[1] 810 kcal (3.4 MJ) is the mean value of the range for energy requirements from 3 months onward (see page 14). – [2] Total long-chain essential fatty acids are taken as 0.68 energy % for the later period of lactation.

the long-chain essential fatty acids has to be taken into account (see page 22).

If the loss during conversion is ignored, the essential fatty acid requirement of the mother would be increased by about 1–2 energy %. Taking the conversion efficiencies into account, the requirement for the parent essential fatty acids in lactation beyond the first hundred days could be between 2 and 4 energy % above the basic essential fatty acid requirements. It is better to express this figure as a range because of the insufficiency of data during this latter period of lactation and the need for the recommendation to reflect the consequent uncertainty.

Maternal undernutrition during lactation

Milk composition varies throughout a single suckling period and during the lactation. The main compositional change is usually in the quantity rather than in the quality of the fat; however, some observations suggest that milk fat is decreased by maternal malnutrition in such a way that the milk cannot provide enough energy or essential fatty acids for the infant (22).

It is recommended that particular attention be given to the mother's extra requirement for energy and essential fatty acids during lactation, as this is the period when the energy requirement is greatest. Indeed, maternal nutrition in pregnancy and lactation requires special priority in the interests of foetal growth, successful lactation, infant nutrition and maternal health.

Requirements in infants and children

INFANTS

The argument that many children have been brought up satisfactorily on cow's milk formulas which contain less than 1% of their energy as essential fatty acids is not convincing, because (a) infants fed on such formulas exhibit significant amounts of eicosatrienoic acid (20:3, n–9) and a triene/tetraene ratio of above 0.2 in their blood lipids (87–89), and (b) show evidence of early vascular pathology in childhood (90). Hence, at 1 energy % as dietary essential fatty acid, the requirements of the infant's normal physiology are possibly not being met. To achieve the composition of long-chain essential fatty acids in blood lipids and a triene/tetraene ratio of below 0.1 comparable to breast-fed infants, an essential fatty acid intake of at least 3 energy % would be required.

Human milk provides essential fatty acids of approximately the same energy % as protein (6%). The long-chain essential fatty acids provide nearly 1 energy % in early lactation. This amount has been neglected because it was thought to be small; it is significant, however, being comparable in amount to certain essential amino acids, and should be taken into account in formulating milk substitutes.

Hence, the ideal recommendation for milk substitutes would be to match the essential fatty acids of human milk from well-nourished mothers with respect to both parent and long-chain essential fatty acids and the balance of n–6 to n–3 families of fatty acids (approximately 5:1).

CHILDREN

Malnutrition

Both protein and structural lipids, with their essential fatty acids, are used for the growth of cell structures in plants and animals. In general, this results in a balance between the availability of protein and essential fatty acids in foods.

It has been customary to think of malnutrition as protein-calorie malnutrition. In practice, diets deficient in protein are also deficient in essential fats. In severe malnutrition, when cell growth is arrested, the associated

36

deficiency of essential fatty acids need not necessarily be obvious, but there is evidence that rehabilitation with diets inadequate in essential fatty acids can precipitate essential fatty acid deficiency (91).

Primary prevention of cardiovascular disease

There is evidence that the blood cholesterol in children at seven years of age in communities with a high risk of coronary heart disease is already significantly higher than in children from low-risk communities (92, 93).

Adolescents from high-risk communities have been found to have significantly more atheromatous lesions than those from low-risk groups (94). Moreover, where dietary patterns change rapidly from those of less developed countries to those of populations with a high risk of atherosclerosis, an increase occurs in the early incidence of morbidity due to cardiovascular disease (95a-e). As nutritional insults are most effective during growth, and as the most active phase in expansion of the vascular surface is childhood, the recommendations for dietary essential fatty acids during infancy and childhood must be taken into account in the prevention of the long-term complications of atherosclerosis, especially with respect to formulas for infant feeding, food preparation for preschool children and school meals. For such purposes, appropriate sources of fats rich in polyunsaturated fatty acids should be used to cover their fatty acid requirements.

6. THE ROLE OF FAT IN THE PREVENTION AND TREATMENT OF CARDIOVASCULAR DISEASES, OBESITY AND DIABETES MELLITUS

Introduction

Cardiovascular diseases, whose incidence is increasing, are the main cause of early death in prosperous population groups throughout the world; obesity and diabetes mellitus increase the risk of their incidence. Infectious diseases and malnutrition are the main causes of morbidity and premature death in unprosperous populations.

Epidemiological data are difficult to interpret. In prosperous populations, in addition to dietary factors, a lack of physical activity, excessive smoking, hypertension, "stress" caused by a competitive social structure and accumulation of toxic environmental substances can all contribute to the progression of cardiovascular disease.

The recommendations of 18 scientific and medical committees on dietary factors and cardiovascular disease (Table 6) are mainly based on the results of a few clinical trials of relatively short duration — short in respect to the life-span of man — and on the known effects of dietary composition on blood lipids.

All the committees recommend that the intake of excess dietary energy, saturated fat and cholesterol should be reduced, and there is international consensus — with the exception of the first report of the Royal Society of New Zealand (1971) and the report of the UK Department of Health and Social Security, Committee on Medical Aspects (DHSS, COMA, 1974) — that the intake of polyunsaturated fatty acids should be increased, preferably to the same level as the intake of saturated fatty acids.

A dietary intake of 30–35% of the energy as fat and a saturated/polyunsaturated fatty acid ratio of 1:1 are in fact generally recommended. As the ratio of saturated fatty acids to monounsaturated fatty acids in most dietary patterns is 1:1, the recommended polyunsaturated fatty acid intake should be about one third of total fatty acid intake — that is, 10–12%.

Cardiovascular diseases

Atherosclerosis is the main nutrition-related cause of cardiovascular diseases. It is a disease of the arteries that, depending on the anatomical location, gradually affects the functioning of heart, brain, kidney, lower extremities or more rarely intestine and spinal cord. Although not usually diagnosed before the age of 40, the onset of this disease occurs in early childhood. Therefore, it has been recently advocated that priority be given to prevention in children (96–98; see also page 37).

From epidemiological evidence (99) and from direct nutritional experiments on laboratory animals (100) and man (99), it is generally concluded that blood lipid concentrations are closely related to the development of atherosclerosis. The type of dietary fat, and specifically the relative proportion of unsaturated to polyunsaturated fatty acids, influences blood lipid levels, the degree of atherosclerosis and the frequency of its complications (100–102). Blood cholesterol levels are also genetically determined (99, 103, 104) and therefore can vary significantly from individual to individual on the same diet.

The body has some capacity to control blood cholesterol levels. Decreasing synthesis occurs when cholesterol is consumed. However, there is strong evidence that these internal controls are unable to maintain low cholesterol levels (101). Changing the cholesterol intake from a high level (700 mg/day) to a low level (100 mg/day) reduces blood cholesterol by about 30 mg/100 ml (0.8 mmol/1) in normal individuals and can substantially reduce risk. In homo- and heterozygous familial hypercholesterolaemia (104) the influence of dietary cholesterol on blood cholesterol is even more pronounced (101, 104, 105). Dietary protein and fibre also affect blood cholesterol levels.

Atherosclerosis is the result of many factors acting on the arterial endothelium and the intima (99, 106). Not only the lipids transported as lipoproteins but also the reactivity of thrombocytes contribute to the progression of the arteriosclerotic lesion. Arterial thrombosis is a major contributor to cardiovascular causes of death, such as acute myocardial infarction and stroke (107).

Arterial thrombosis

The favourable influence of diets high in linoleic acid (18:2, n–6) and low in saturated fat on the prevention or regression of atherosclerotic disease is commonly explained by their blood-cholesterol-lowering effect (100–102). However, the saturated fatty acids — especially palmitic (16:0) and stearic (18:0) acids — increase the thrombotic tendency of blood platelets, whereas linoleic acid (18:2, n–6) diminishes that tendency, thereby significantly reducing arterial thrombus formation. These dietary effects have been confirmed in several clinical studies (108–112). The favourable effect of linoleic acid can be explained by its influence on prostaglandin metabolism (108).

TABLE 6. – RECOMMENDATIONS OF 18 SCIENTIFIC AND MEDICAL COMMITTEES ON DIETARY FATS AND CORONARY HEART DISEASE [1]

Country and committee	General population (GP), high-risk group (HR)	Fat content of total energy (%)	Increased PUFA [2]	PUFA-SAFA [3] ratio	Daily dietary cholesterol (mg)	Reduction of sugar	Labelling of fat content of foods
Norway, Sweden & Finland, 1968	GP	25–35			–		Yes
United States, 1970 Inter-Society	GP	<35	Yes	1.0	<300	Yes	Yes
	HR						
New Zealand, 1971 Heart Foundation	GP	35	Yes	1.0	300–600	No	Yes
	HR	35	Yes	1.0	300–600	No	Yes
New Zealand, 1971 Royal Society	GP	Avoid excess saturated fat	No		Reduce		–
	HR		Yes		Reduce		–
New Zealand, 1976 Royal Society	GP	Decrease saturated fat					
United States, 1972 American Health Foundation	GP	35	Yes	1.0	300	Yes	Yes
United States, 1972 American Medical Association	HR	Substantial decrease in saturated fat	Yes		Reduce		Yes
International Society of Cardiology, 1973	HR	<30	Yes	>1.0	<300		Yes
United States, 1973 American Heart Association	GP	35	Yes	1.0	300		Yes

TABLE 6. – RECOMMENDATIONS OF 18 SCIENTIFIC AND MEDICAL COMMITTEES ON DIETARY FATS AND CORONARY HEART DISEASE [1] (concluded)

Country and committee	General population (GP), high-risk group (HR)	Fat content of total energy (%)	Increased PUFA [2]	PUFA-SAFA [3] ratio	Daily dietary cholesterol (mg)	Reduction of sugar	Labelling of fat content of foods
The Netherlands, 1973	GP	35	Yes	1.0	250–300	Yes	Yes
United States, 1973 White House Conference	GP	35	Yes	–	300	–	Yes
Australia, 1974 National Heart Foundation ..	GP HR	30–35	Yes	1.5	<300	– Yes	–
United Kingdom, 1974 DHSS, COMA report	GP	Reduce total fat, esp. saturated	No	–	–	Yes	–
Germany (F.R.), 1975	GP	Reduce saturated fat	Yes	–	300	–	–
Australia, 1975 Academy of Science	GP	35	Yes	1.0	<350	Yes	Yes
United Kingdom, 1976 Royal College of Physicians & British Cardiac Society [4] ...	GP	Toward 35	Yes	–	Reduce	Yes	Yes
Norway, 1976 Ministry of Agriculture	GP	35	Yes	Increase	–	Yes	Yes
Canada, 1976 Dept. of Health and Welfare	GP HR	30–35 30–35	Yes Yes	– –	400 400	Yes Yes	Yes Yes
United States, 1977 Senate Committee	GP HR	30 30	Yes Yes	1.0 1.0	300 300	Yes Yes	– –

[1] From Turner and Ball (1977), *Postgraduate Medical Journal*. – [2] PUFA = polyunsaturated fatty acids. – [3] SAFA = saturated fatty acids. –
[4] Not official committee of the UK.

41

Hypertension

Genetic predisposition, prolonged intake of a high-sodium diet and obesity all contribute to a high incidence of hypertension (113). Recent studies in rats have shown that increased dietary linoleic acid (18:2, n-6) counteracts salt-induced hypertension (114–116). These results can be explained on the basis of changes in prostaglandin metabolism (114, 117–119). These data obtained with rats are strengthened by two pilot studies with humans (120, 121), but they need further confirmation.

Obesity

Obesity is a risk factor in cardiovascular disease because it results in hypertension and maturity-onset diabetes. The prevention and therapy of obesity are difficult as there exists in many individuals a genetic predisposition to become obese, which for evident reasons cannot be efficiently corrected. Therapy is also complicated by strong psychological factors leading for a variety of reasons to overeating. If this is also accompanied by a lack of exercise and an abundant supply of relatively low-cost, attractive, ready-to-eat foods, it is not too surprising that obesity has become one of the major health problems (122).

Many dietary measures are based on the assumption that a change in the ratio of nutrients induces a reduction of food intake. Carbohydrates and fats are the nutrients most involved because they are the main energy sources; the possibilities of increasing protein intake are very limited because of cost and the danger of overloading kidney function.

As has already been stated, it is difficult to isolate physiological factors in the diet from emotional and behavioural factors which normally influence food intake. A recent short-term investigation (123) has shown that even wide variations in the carbohydrate/fat ratio do not influence voluntary food intake. More research is required to determine whether this is also true in experiments of longer duration.

It is probably more important in obesity prevention and therapy to concentrate on reducing the intake of empty calories, such as sugar, alcohol, and saturated and monounsaturated fatty acids, in order to guarantee a sufficient intake of foods that are adequate in protein, EFAS, vitamins and minerals and contain sufficient indigestible material to improve intestinal function. Total energy intake should maintain ideal body weight and composition in adults and optimize growth rates and vital functions in children.

Diabetes mellitus

The increasing worldwide incidence of diabetes mellitus is associated with higher average life expectancy, improved standard of living and increased survival rate of young diabetics to the reproductive age. Diabetes mellitus is assumed to have a hereditary component which becomes manifest because of obesity, multiple pregnancies or infections (124–126).

No existing classification of diabetes mellitus is satisfactory. There is still no agreement as to whether it should be classified according to the insulin secretory capacity of the pancreas or on the basis of impaired glucose tolerance. The determination of its real incidence is very difficult because of its insidious onset in many cases of obesity. Another difficulty is the disappearance of the chemical symptoms when the patient is on a successful slimming diet.

Vascular disorders, macro- and micro-angiopathy, occur frequently at an early stage in diabetes mellitus. A recent review of the relationship between abnormal circulating insulin levels and atherosclerosis concluded that high levels of circulating insulin contribute to the development of atherosclerosis (127). This may explain why the long-term results of treatment of diabetes mellitus are so disappointing.

The dietary strategy for the two main types of diabetes mellitus has been reviewed recently (125, 128, 129). Most therapies concentrate on the control of hyperglycaemia; however, in diabetes mellitus, hyperlipidaemia is always present and should be treated in the same way as hyperlipidaemias from other causes. A well-controlled clinical experiment on obese, non-insulin-requiring diabetics (125) has demonstrated that even without weight reduction, an isocaloric diet high in linoleic acid (about 25 energy %) can significantly lower blood cholesterol, fasting and nonfasting blood triglycerides, blood glucose and insulin concentration over a period of ten days. The tentative nature of this experiment does not allow definite conclusions, and further experiments along these lines are necessary.

An excess of food energy is laid down as fat, especially in the presence of insulin. Before insulin came into use, fat was the main source of energy for the diabetic. Since that time the allowed amount of carbohydrate has steadily been increased (130–131).

Until now, no attention has been paid to the quality of the dietary fat. In practice, diets for diabetics were high in saturated fatty acids and cholesterol, because butter, cream and eggs were considered advantageous for the diabetic patient. The positive atherogenicity of these fats (125, 132) may explain to a great extent the poor long-term results of diabetes therapy. Almost all investigations suffer from the restricted criteria used, as only some measures of carbohydrate metabolism have been studied, namely glycaemia and glycosuria. Furthermore, no sharp distinction is made between macro- and micro-angiopathy. Diabetic macro-angiopathy is not different from atherosclerosis without diabetes, but diabetic micro-angiopathy is almost specific for diabetes. The latter complication can be favourably influenced by a strict control of diabetes (132), whereas the prevention of atherosclerosis does not differ from that in nondiabetic individuals.

Conclusions

Hypocaloric diets will induce significant decreases in body weight and blood cholesterol, triglyceride and insulin levels, and will normalize most cases of maturity-onset diabetes. After ideal body weight is reached, a normal maintenance diet should be used.

Food habits in population groups with a high incidence of athero-sclerosis, obesity and maturity-onset diabetes are such that it will be difficult to achieve a reduction in fat intake below 30 energy %. Furthermore, in the commonly consumed food products the invisible fat is mostly saturated, and the EFAS have to come mainly from visible fat sources. For these reasons the generally recommended diet for the prevention of atheroclerosis should contain energy to maintain ideal body weight, 10–15 energy % of protein, 30–35 energy % of fat, with less than one third saturated fatty acids and at least one third linoleic acid (18:2, n-6). It should be low in refined sugars and alcohol and contain less than 300 mg of cholesterol per day (Table 6).

There is good evidence from studies on animals and humans that such diets will significantly decrease two main risk factors for atherosclerosis: (i) blood lipoproteins carrying cholesterol and triglycerides; and (ii) thrombotic tendency of blood platelets.

Furthermore, there are indications that such diets may have preventive and curative effects in sodium-induced hypertension and may normalize carbohydrate metabolism in maturity-onset diabetes.

44

7. EFFECTS OF PROCESSING ON THE NUTRITIVE VALUE OF FATS AND OILS USED IN HUMAN NUTRITION

Introduction

Until comparatively recent times, edible oils and fats were extracted locally by mechanical operations, with or without the application of moisture and external heat, and were used in unrefined form. This practice is still widespread in many countries and, apart from alterations caused by release of free fatty acids or rancidity, all nutrients naturally present remain in the product. The major vegetable oils traditionally consumed in many countries in a clean but unrefined form are groundnut, coconut, rapeseed, mustardseed, palm, olive and sesameseed oils. Fats and oils of animal origin include tallow, lard and oils from marine mammals and fish.

For about fifty years, vegetable fats and oils have also been obtained by more efficient mechanical expression and by solvent extraction. Furthermore, they are subjected to technological processes to make them as bland and colourless as possible. The refining techniques consist of washing, alkali refining, bleaching and deodorization. The resultant oils and fats may be further processed by hydrogenation, randomization and winterization for different food uses. Figures 3 and 4 show the steps commonly used in oil processing.

Most vegetable oils used for human food are relatively high in polyunsaturated fatty acids, primarily linoleic acid (18:2, n–6), but in some oils small amounts of α-linolenic acid (18:3, n–3) are also present. These fatty acids are susceptible to autoxidation if not properly protected by adequate antioxidants. Vegetable oils naturally contain compounds of the vitamin E family, tocopherols and tocotrienols, which are effective antioxidants in stabilizing these oils under normal storage conditions. If oils are overheated or re-used excessively for deep-fat frying of foods, loss of vitamin E and formation of oxidized and polymerized products occur. Early studies with animals showed that these products can be toxic, raising questions of possible adverse effects of overheated oils in human nutrition. Subsequent investigations of the nutritional effects of used cooking oils have indicated that under practical dietary conditions these oils have no detrimental effects and that long-term possibilities of toxic manifestations are remote (132a).

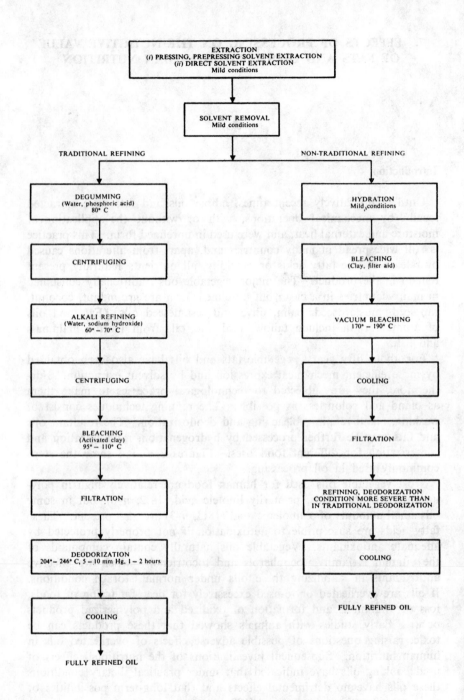

FIGURE 3. Steps in preparing an edible oil.

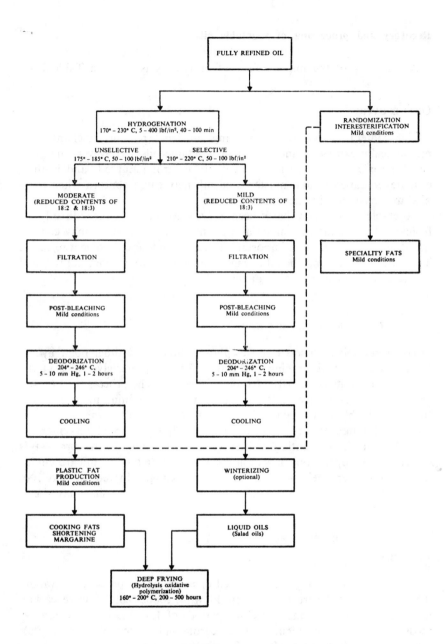

FIGURE 4. Further transformation of edible oils.

Recovery and processing of vegetable oils

A summary of the major effects of processing is given in Table 7.

OIL RECOVERY

The content of naturally occurring nutrients remains unchanged in mechanically expressed and unrefined vegetable oils. However, the presence of toxic materials, such as aflatoxin in groundnut oils and isothiocyanates in rapeseed and mustardseed oil, may cause concern when these oils are consumed in the unrefined form.

Vegetable oils which have been solvent-extracted, either directly or from residues of the raw material after mechanical pressing, may contain traces of solvents or, more important, traces of undesirable solvent residues. The process of heating the oil to high temperatures to ensure total removal of these substances may also damage the oil.

DEGUMMING AND ALKALI REFINING

The degumming process removes phospholipids and other polar hydratable lipids. Alkali refining has little effect on the triglycerides in the oil and thus on its principal nutritional function. The process is employed to remove the free fatty acids. In addition, alkali refining removes nutritionally valuable constituents, such as carotenoids (often mostly β-carotene). Although the removal of water-binding phospholipids may be advantageous in preventing spattering and browning if the product is used for frying operations, it is desirable to minimize the loss of carotenoids and to consider their addition after processing. In red palm oil, an important source of carotene in certain populations, refining may therefore not be desirable.

BLEACHING

Bleaching consists of treating refined oils with small proportions (about 0.5%) of activated earths, often mixed with about 0.05% active carbon at temperatures of around 100°C for periods of 15–30 minutes, to remove most of the remaining pigments (e.g., carotenoids, chlorophyll, gossypol); however, the acidic nature of most bleaching earths gives rise to measurable quantities of conjugated fatty acids derived from the polyunsaturated fatty acids present. Peroxidized fatty acids also break down to yield conjugated compounds. The nutritional significance of the conjugated

TABLE 7. – EFFECTS OF PROCESSING VEGETABLE OILS

Process	Fat components altered/added	Components removed/reduced
Solvent extraction	Residual solvents in small amounts Minor modification of the oils if heating is excessive	
Degumming		Hydratable non-oil materials, mostly carbohydrates and proteins, partially removed Hydratable non-glyceridic lipids, such as phospholipids, partially removed Chlorophyll partially removed, especially if phosphoric acid is employed
Alkali refining		Free fatty acids and other materials removed Residual phospholipids removed Proteinaceous materials reduced in quantity Colouring matter reduced in quantity
Bleaching	Conjugated acids formed and peroxides destroyed	Carotenoids removed Chlorophyll and its decomposition products removed Gossypol-like pigments removed Toxic agents, such as polycyclic aromatic hydrocarbons, removed (if carbon is used in quantity)
Deodorization	Formation of geometrical isomers in sensitive acids Formation of linear and cyclic dimers/polymers	Free fatty acids, peroxide decomposition products, colour bodies and their decomposition products eliminated Sterols and sterol esters reduced in quantity Tocopherols reduced in quantity Pesticide residues and mycotoxins removed totally
Hydrogenation	Partial saturation Formation of positional and geometric isomers Formation of linear and cyclic dimers/polymers	Essential fatty acids reduced in quantity
Winterization	Enhancement of unsaturated triglycerides	Higher-melting triglycerides removed
Randomization & interesterification	Rearrangement of triglycerides to a more random distribution	

49

acids has not yet been clearly defined. Transformation of sterols into materials with unknown biological properties is also suspected to occur during bleaching.

During the process of vacuum bleaching, when temperatures are as high as 170°–190°C, and large quantities of acid-activated clay are used, positional and geometric isomers are produced from the more reactive fatty acids. Active carbon can remove phenanthrenes, α-benzpyrenes and similar compounds when these are present.

DEODORIZATION

The passage of steam through layers of oil held in trays under vacuum at temperatures of about 250°C strips the oil of traces of free fatty acids, volatile fat oxidation breakdown products and other odoriferous compounds. At the same time, other effects occur, such as the partial removal of both free and esterified sterols and tocopherols. Nevertheless, the simultaneous removal of all pesticide and organochlorine residues and of mycotoxins is clearly beneficial.

During deodorization the tocopherol content of the oil is frequently reduced by one third. Since vegetable oils, especially those containing essential fatty acids, are good dietary sources of tocopherols, such losses could be detrimental, although in practice there is rarely a recognizable dietary shortage of vitamin E even in the diets of low-income populations.

The high temperatures used in the deodorization process cause limited isomerization by changing the natural cis-trans configurations in both linoleic (18:2, n–6) and α-linolenic (18:3, n–3) acids. In fact, the degree of isomerization is a sensitive index of the degree of undesirable changes in the oil. The formation of conjugated acids of cyclic monomers through intramolecular bonding and of polymers through intermolecular bonding is likely to occur. New deodorization techniques, in which trays and towers are replaced by thin films of oil through which steam is blown, greatly reduce residence time and are believed to produce only a fraction of the changes occurring in conventional cascade-type or bubble-tray equipment. Such technological developments should be encouraged.

In unrefined oils of exceptionally good quality, direct deodorization is now being used for removal of free fatty acids. The step of alkali refining after hydration and vacuum bleaching is omitted. The effects of such physical refining on oils containing linoleic (18:2, n–6) and α-linolenic (18:3, n–3) acids require further study, as deodorization is conducted at even higher temperatures and over longer periods of time than with the conventional procedure.

50

Further transformation

HYDROGENATION

Slight hydrogenation is used to increase the stability of certain fatty materials by selective reduction of the level of α-linolenic acid (18:3, *n*–3). To a much greater extent it is used for less selective conversion of large quantities of liquid oils into semisolid fats which are eaten as such or after further processing. Partial hydrogenation results in extensive changes in the fatty acids of triglycerides, reduces the carotenoid pigments and lightens the colour, but does not affect tocopherols.

Saturation of all the unsaturated bonds in one triglyceride molecule or in one molecule of fatty acid is rarely the major effect of partial hydrogenation. Extensive shifts of the unsaturated bonds occur in both polyunsaturated and monounsaturated acids, yielding a wide range of both positional and geometric isomers with the same number of, or fewer, unsaturated bonds as the original fatty acids. Conjugated materials of complex nature are known to be produced, and cyclic monomers and intramolecular linear dimers are also generated. A loss of essential fatty acids (EFAS) is axiomatic in hydrogenation.

Fatty acids with trans configurations occur in proportions of from 5% to 45% in commercial hydrogenated fat products. The feeding of such fats to animals such as rats and swine, even for several generations, has shown no undesirable effects. Nutritional studies comparing hydrogenated oils with their starting materials have shown no particular differences if the need for EFAS and other nutrients lost during hydrogenation is met (132b,c).

Research is currently being conducted on the effects of isomeric fatty acids on cellular membrane structures and cellular functions.

WINTERIZATION

The process of winterization removes higher-melting triglycerides from a chilled oil and produces a liquid oil that remains clear at refrigerator temperatures. If employed in the processing of oils such as cottonseed oil or of partially hydrogenated materials containing triglycerides rich in saturated or trans fatty acids, the removal of these compounds increases the proportion of the unsaturated fatty acids in the winterized product and can therefore be considered as nutritionally beneficial. The higher-melting triglycerides removed from nonhydrogenated oils are suitable for use as the solid fat matrix in margarines and shortening. If derived from partially hydrogenated oils, this fraction of higher-melting triglycerides may also include trans acids.

51

During this process, conducted under dry oxygen-free conditions at moderate or low temperatures, fatty acids in the triglyceride molecules are rearranged to assume a more random distribution. Randomization of a single oil generally changes its consistency and raises its melting point. When two oils are present, the process is called interesterification. A common application of this process is to produce a plastic fat from a polyunsaturated liquid oil interesterified with a smaller amount of fully saturated fat. The nutritional value of any linoleic acid (18:2, *n*–6) present has been shown experimentally to be unimpaired (132d).

Toxic substances in vegetable oils

ENDOGENOUS SUBSTANCES

Cyclopropenoid acids are characteristic of plants of the order *Malvales*. Crude cottonseed oils and kapokseed oil contain 1–2% and about 24%, respectively, of total cyclopropenoid acids, specifically malvalic and sterculic acids (133). Cocoa butter is free of these acids, although the cocoa tree belongs to the same botanical order. Alkali-refining of cottonseed oil does not reduce the content of cyclopropenoid fatty acids markedly, but deodorization reduces it severalfold, as does partial hydrogenation. Residual levels of cyclopropenoid fatty acids in fully refined cottonseed oil are sufficiently low to avoid adverse effects on man. Refined groundnut, coconut, soybean and herring oils have been investigated and found free of nitrogenous substances thought to be allergenic (134).

Oxidized fat has been shown to be toxic; however, soybean oil with a peroxide value as high as 100 did not induce obvious toxic symptoms when fed to rats at 20 energy % of the diet (135). Peroxide values of this level do not occur under normal processing. Although peroxidation is a potential hazard to be avoided, it is not probable in this instance. Moreover, deodorization destroys peroxides, and in any case, fats containing even 10 milliequivalents of peroxide per gram are unpalatable to most consumers.

EXOGENOUS MATERIALS

Organochlorine compounds are now ubiquitous, and pesticide residues of this type, as well as polychlorinated biphenyl compounds, are often found in unrefined vegetable oils at levels between three and ten times their detectable limits (136). Marine oils contain these materials, and they can also be found in ruminant fats. Current refining practices reduce the levels of these compounds in refined vegetable oils to insignificant proportions.

Pyrolysis of chlorinated phenols can yield chlorinated dibenzo-p-dioxin and its isomers, all of which produce hydropericardial symptoms. The reaction conditions for their formation are likely to occur during vegetable oil processing. As the polarity and molecular weights of these compounds do not differ markedly from those of DDT, it can be expected that the deodorization process will also remove such materials. The polycyclic aromatic hydrocarbons anthracene and phenanthrene occur naturally in palm oil which also contains carotenoid pigments. Palm oil is now sometimes refined by the non-traditional "physical refining" process, which employs relatively high temperatures (220°–270°C). Concern that carotenoid pigments would thereby be cyclized to produce increased quantities of polycyclic aromatic hydrocarbons has not been substantiated, as the level of polycyclic aromatic hydrocarbons in palm oil decreases after such refining (137).

Deep frying operations

Oils commonly used in deep frying processes are vegetable oils, such as groundnut, sunflowerseed, soybean and rapeseed oils to which permitted chemical antioxidants may have been added. Partially hydrogenated (semisolid) vegetable oils, vegetable oils with a high content of saturated fatty acids (coconut oil, palm oil) or animal fats are seldom used as their appearance and palatability on cooling are not attractive to the consumer.

Deep frying consists of the immersion of food in hot fats or oils. Some oil (pick-up oil) penetrates and cooks the outer layers of the food or breading, but oil transfer to the interior of the product is minimal. Surplus oil is drained off into the main body of oil, where pieces of the product and breading may also accumulate. In some operations, fresh oil is frequently added to make up for lost pick-up oil when processing is continuous, so that the peroxides and polymers formed are thus constantly diluted and removed. An important part of quality control is the monitoring of peroxide values in the oil used. In batch operations in industry, institutions, food services and the home, polymer build-up in frying oil is a serious matter. Some polymers are not absorbed by the body and are thus simply wasteful in energy terms, but other carbon-oxygen linked materials, or cyclic products, are likely to be deleterious to health and require careful study. Pick-up oil has been shown to contain residual tocopherol, which contributes to the total dietary intake of tocopherol.

Conclusions

Oil refining operations reduce the levels of certain nutrients, which could be of specific concern where the unrefined oil is the principal source of the nutrient. In some instances, undesirable components are also removed, with consequent improvement in the quality of the oil. Deodorization produces appreciable quantities of isomers of linoleic acid (18:2, *n*–6) when unnecessarily severe conditions are applied. The physiological significance of these isomers should be further studied. The severity of deodorization conditions must be reduced, especially when physical refining is applied to oils containing linoleic acid (18:2, *n*–6). New and less drastic processes need to be developed.

The nature of the by-product artefacts of the hydrogenation and deodorization processes should be established and their biological significance carefully examined. More work on the biochemical effects of polymers is advocated. There is also a need for extensive research on the nature and nutritional effects of by-products developed during fat frying.

8. SPECIAL CONSIDERATIONS

Health implications of brassica-derived oils

Oils derived from seeds of various *Brassica* spp., such as rapeseed oil and mustardseed oil, are produced and consumed in many countries. The most characteristic feature of these oils is the presence of erucic acid (cis-Δ13-docosenoic acid; 22:1, *n*–9), amounting to 20–55% of the total fatty acids. In addition, these oils contain about 10% 11-eicosenoic acid (20:1, *n*–9). These two long-chain fatty acids are not present in appreciable amounts in other vegetable oils used for human consumption. Through plant breeding the content of erucic acid (22:1, *n*–9) and 11-eicosenoic acid (20:1, *n*–9) has been lowered to close to zero in some varieties of rapeseed (see also Chapter 10). Oils with a high level of erucic acid (22:1, *n*–9) contain a low proportion of oleic acid (18:1, *n*–9); as the erucic acid content decreases, that of oleic acid increases, while the proportions of the other fatty acids vary only slightly. Brassicasterol is a characteristic constituent of brassica oils and can be used for identification of them. The seeds also contain sulphur compounds — the glucosinolates.

Reports published since the 1940s have revealed that feeding large amounts of rapeseed oil high in erucic acid (22:1, *n*–9) to laboratory animals causes growth retardation and changes in the heart, adrenals and liver. However, this observation did not bring about any action regarding human consumption until early in the 1970s.

Brassica oils constitute an important source of vegetable oils, preceded only by soybean, sunflowerseed, groundnut, cottonseed and palm oils (see Table 14, page 74). The main producers of rapeseed are India, Canada, China, some European countries, Pakistan and Bangladesh. Rapeseed and rapeseed oil are mainly exported from Canada and Europe; the main importing countries without domestic production are Japan and the North African countries (Tables 8 and 9).

In several countries with populations consuming diets with a high proportion of fat, production of rapeseed oil expanded rapidly from the 1940s onward. In those countries rapeseed oil can be considered an untraditional source of dietary energy. In countries such as India and China, however, rapeseed and rapeseed oil have a long tradition as foods; there production has increased less.

TABLE 8. – PRODUCTION/IMPORT/EXPORT OF RAPESEED BY MAJOR COUNTRIES, 1975
(Thousand metric tons)

Production		Export [1]		Import [1]	
WORLD	8 121	WORLD	1 048	WORLD	1 127
India	2 211	Canada	734	Japan	669
Canada	1 635	Sweden	118	Germany, F.R.	130
China	[2] 1 254	Denmark	62	France	55
Poland	700	France	48	Netherlands	48
France	532	Poland	[3] 30	United Kingdom	48
Sweden	332	Germany, F.R.	12	Bangladesh	[3] 43
Pakistan	248	Hungary	[3] 11	Algeria	[3] 40
Bangladesh	[3] 110				

SOURCES: *FAO production yearbook, 1975; FAO trade yearbook, 1975.*
[1] Includes mustardseed. – [2] FAO estimate. – [3] Unofficial.

TABLE 9. – IMPORT/EXPORT OF RAPESEED AND MUSTARDSEED OILS BY MAJOR COUNTRIES AND TERRITORIES, 1975
(Thousand metric tons)

Export		Import	
WORLD	353	WORLD	277
France	118	Morocco	84
Germany, F.R.	64	Algeria	[1] 25
Poland	[1] 52	Hong Kong	[1] 24
Sweden	39	Germany, F.R.	19
Netherlands	33	Japan	15
Canada	20	Italy	14

SOURCES: *FAO production yearbook, 1975; FAO trade yearbook, 1975.*
[1] Unofficial.

The amount of fat consumed varies from one region to another, and what may be a health implication in one part of the world is not necessarily such in another. The average consumption of fats in different countries is reported in Chapter 9.

Observations in regions of India where the diet contains unrefined brassica oils indicated that the extent of lipidosis and necrosis in human hearts was no different from that in other populations consuming groundnut and sesameseed oils (138).

STUDIES ON RAPESEED OIL HIGH IN ERUCIC ACID

The main results of three extensive reviews of the nutritional properties of rapeseed oil (139–141) are shown in Table 10.

Brassica oils that are high in erucic acid (22:1, n–9) cause retarded growth in some experimental animals. Various organs are adversely affected morphologically, biochemically and functionally. The heart and red skeletal muscle of young rats showed intracellular fat accumulation after administration of rapeseed oil; with continued feeding, the amount of fat in the heart regressed, but the contractility of the heart muscle was impaired (188). Little is known about the mechanism of fat regression from heart and skeletal muscles. Concomitant with fat accumulation, a decrease of the glycogen stores in the heart was found, indicative of a shift in metabolism. Other chemical findings were changes in the proportions of different phospholipids and of the fatty acid composition of mitochondrial membranes.

Later myocardial changes were characterized by cellular infiltration, death of heart muscle cells and replacement of these by scar tissue. These lesions did not occur in the rat when rapeseed oil was removed from the diet after one week. A sex difference in the response to rapeseed oil has been reported, especially regarding changes in the heart, which were more severe in the male rat. There is generally close agreement between different laboratories on the effects caused by oils high in erucic acid.

Synthetic triglycerides containing erucic acid also induced fat accumulation and long-term lesions in the hearts of rats. Isomers of erucic acid present in partially hydrogenated rapeseed oil produced cardiac lipidosis. This condition has also been observed in such species as gerbils, rabbits, guinea pigs, monkeys and ducklings when fed rapeseed oil with a high erucic acid content. The degree and pattern of occurrence varied among species. There was agreement in three studies on monkeys (squirrel, macaque and cynomolgus monkeys) that brassica oils high in erucic acid caused lipidosis (141). In humans fed high erucic acid rapeseed oil the platelet count was greatly reduced (189).

Organ or site	Animal	Dietary oil	Effect	References
Body fat	Rat	Rapeseed oil	Ovary and adrenal fat most influenced	142–148
	Swine	Rapeseed oil	Plasma and adipose tissue fat influenced	149
			Erucic acid mainly incorporated in triglycerides and in smaller amounts in phospholipids, with the exception of adrenals and ovaries, where erucic acid is incorporated mainly in the cholesterol ester fraction	146, 150–153
				144, 154–156
Milk	Rat	Rapeseed oil	Eicosenoic acid and erucic acid present in the milk	151, 157
Adrenals	Rat	Rapeseed oil	Enlarged and contained more fat	154, 156, 158–161
			During cold stress ($+ 4^{\circ}$C) cholesteryl erucate less efficiently utilized for the synthesis of steroid hormones, lower plasma corticosterone level	162
			Low rat survival rates in the cold	163–164
Reproduction	Rat	Rapeseed oil	Mortality of the offspring high due to deficient mammary development and lactation in the mother	165
		Rapeseed oil Maize oil	Lower weanling weights in young rats fed rapeseed oil than in rats fed maize oil	166
		Rapeseed oil	Fewer and smaller offspring	157
Blood	Guinea pig Chicken	Rapeseed oil	Tendency to hypercholesterolaemia	175

Organ or site	Animal	Dietary oil	Effect	References
Blood	Rabbit	Rapeseed oil	Influence on blood cholesterol	161, 175
	Duckling	Rapeseed oil	Increased haematocrit and reticulocyte count	170
Liver	Rat	Rapeseed oil	No histological lesions after short time; after 1–2 years, indication of fatty infiltration and degeneration in central parts of lobes	160–161, 167–169
	Duckling	Rapeseed oil at 30 energy %	Cirrhotic changes after three weeks	170
	Duckling Guinea pig	Isocaloric oil + erucic acid	With increased level of dietary palmitic acid, fewer cases of liver cirrhosis	171–172
	Duckling Chicken Pig	Rapeseed oil	Increased erythropoesis in the liver	169, 171, 173
Spleen	Duckling Guinea pig	Rapeseed oil at 30 energy %	Atrophy of the red pulp, lipidosis, increased erythropoesis	171
	Guinea pig	Rapeseed oil at 50 energy %	Hypertrophic spleen with enlarged fat-infiltrated red pulp, intensive erythropoesis	169
Kidney	Rat	Rapeseed oil	Increased kidney weight, nephrosis characterized by vacuolation of the tubular epithelium, tubular dilatation, focal connective tissue proliferation	159–161
	Female rat	Rapeseed oil	Renal concentration capacity lowered	174
Skeletal muscles	Rat	Rapeseed oil at 60 energy %	Reversible fatty infiltration	159–161
	Duckling	Rapeseed oil at 30 energy %	Fatty accumulation, oedema, disintegration of the muscle fibres, cell infiltration	170

Organ or site	Animal	Dietary oil	Effect	References
Heart	Growing rat	Rapeseed oil	Intracellular lipidosis, histiocytic infiltration, finally fibrosis	159, 161, 176–178, 186–187
		Rapeseed oil at 30 energy %	Dose-related lipidosis	178
		Rapeseed oil at 20 energy %	Some abnormal accumulation of fat	177
			Lipidosis of the myocardium that never disappears completely	160, 176–177
	Adult rat	Rapeseed oil	Milder lipidosis	160, 179, 180
	Rat Duckling Guinea pig Rabbit Gerbil Miniature pig Piglet Squirrel monkey	Rapeseed oil	Lipidosis of the heart muscle	161, 170–171, 180
	Duckling	Rapeseed oil	Severe hydropericardium	170
	Rat	Rapeseed oil	Focal or diffuse infiltrations of mononuclear cells, histiocytes proliferation of fibroblasts	160
			Fibrosis	179
			Pathological changes	159, 160, 170, 178
		Docosenoic acid	Lipidosis, degenerative lesions in the myocardium	177, 181
		Eicosenoic acid	Fat droplets	182
		Erucic or cetoleic acid	Appreciably greater accumulation of myocardial lipids	182
		Rapeseed oil	Accumulation of triglycerides in the heart	183–185

It was apparent that rapeseed oil high in erucic acid had an unusually slow rate of absorption in the rat (190) and that the digestibility was about 80%. Both the slow absorption and the low digestibility were attributed to the presence of erucic acid, which occupies positions 1 and 3 in the triglycerides of rapeseed oil. After interesterification, which randomly distributes the fatty acids in all three positions of the triglycerides, erucic acid was better absorbed by the rat.

In humans an average digestion of rapeseed oil as high as 98.8% was reported as early as 1918 (191) and was later confirmed. For erucic acid an absorption of 99% was reported. Dietary erucic acid digestion and transport in the human being were normal. However, incorporation of erucic acid in different lipid classes of chylomicrons and very low density lipoproteins was somewhat different from that of oleic (18:1, n-9) and palmitic (16:0) acids.

MITOCHONDRIA

Oxidation

Feeding of dietary rapeseed oil with a high content of erucic acid (22:1, n-9) resulted in fat accumulation in the hearts of different species of experimental animals. As the deviations in fat metabolism were primarily observed in heart and skeletal muscle, in which a major function of the fatty acids is to supply energy to the muscle cells, it appeared that erucic acid was less efficiently oxidized.

It has been suggested (192) that the inhibitory effect of erucic acid might be exerted on any one of the following steps in the mitochondria: fatty acid activation; acyl-CoA transfer across the mitochondrial inner membrane; beta-oxidation of the activated fatty acid to acetyl-CoA; and, finally, complete oxidation of active acetate to carbon dioxide and water. Studies on the ability of mitochondria isolated from rat hearts to oxidize substrates and to synthesize adenosine triphosphate (ATP) have led to considerable controversy. A depressed production of energy first reported (176) was not subsequently confirmed.

The translocation of erucic acid through the mitochondrial membrane involved its carnitine derivative, but no difference in the relative amounts of free carnitine to acyl carnitine in the rat heart was found. It was also reported that oxygen uptake was lower in the presence of erucoyl carnitine than with palmitoyl carnitine, suggesting that the presence of erucic acid had an inhibitory effect on the beta-oxidation of other fatty acids, which could explain the accumulation of triglycerides.

The *in vitro* oxidation of palmitoyl carnitine was reduced by more than 50% even with levels of erucic acid as low as 1.4% in the diet. It was reported that the activity of acyl-CoA-dehydrogenase progressively decreased from oleoyl-CoA to eicosenoyl-CoA to erucoyl-CoA. It was found that erucoyl carnitine competitively inhibited the oxidation of other acyl carnitines in the heart mitochondria. Furthermore, the carnitine esters of the isomers of erucic, cetoleic (22:1, *n*-11) and brassidic (trans 22:1, *n*-9) acids, which are formed during hydrogenation, were reported to undergo both intramitochondrial-CoA acylation and beta-oxidation at the same slow rate as erucoyl carnitine (193–195).

Incorporation of erucic acid into membrane phospholipids

At high dietary levels of erucic acid (22:1, *n*-9), the cardiac triglycerides contained over 50% erucic acid and the phospholipids about 7%. Another study reported that erucic acid constituted 2.5% of the fatty acids of the phospholipid fraction. Erucic acid was found to be incorporated into the cardiolipin fraction of rat heart mitochondria at the expense of linoleic acid (18:2, *n*-6), which suggested that erucic acid as a constituent of cardiolipin in the inner mitochondrial membrane might influence energy production (153).

Studies of low erucic acid brassica oils

Body and organ weights

Rapeseed oil low in erucic acid permitted the same growth in rats as other fats and oils (196); also food intakes were the same as in the control animals. Growth- and appetite-depressing effects attributed to the presence of erucic acid were not present (196a). It was also found that the growth rate of male and female rats fed rapeseed oil with 1% erucic acid as 30 energy % did not differ from that of control animals receiving groundnut oil (197). The feed efficiency of the diet containing oil low in erucic acid was the same as the efficiency of the control diet. From a study with ducklings it was concluded that there was no significant difference in growth rate when these animals were given 50 energy % as rapeseed oil containing 8.5% erucic acid from that of the control animals given 50 energy % sunflowerseed oil. No influence on growth rate was reported in rats when low erucic acid rapeseed oil was supplemented with palmitic acid (16:0), whereas high erucic acid rapeseed oil needed supplementation.

The weights of heart, spleen, pancreas, testes and adrenals in the rat were normal when low erucic acid rapeseed oil was fed as 30% of the energy (196). Inconsistent reports mention, however, an increase in the weights of the liver and kidneys. In ducklings fed low erucic acid rapeseed oil normal weights of pancreas, spleen, liver, kidneys and heart have been reported.

Histopathology

Histologically detectable moderate lipidosis was reported with about 2% of the energy as erucic acid and slight lipidosis at a level of about 0.8 energy % (186). Intracellular deposition of lipid droplets was consistently reported when high erucic acid rapeseed oils were fed. It was also well established that this deposition was related to the dietary level of erucic acid. Apart from effects of low erucic acid rapeseed oils on the heart, no abnormal alterations have been observed in any organ.

Long-term lesions

Cellular infiltrations, lysis of heart muscle fibres, and fibrosis were observed in male rats fed low erucic acid rapeseed oil as 30% of energy; female rats showed only a slight response to this oil (197). Reports also indicate that variations in response occur in different strains of rats. Other studies with 40% energy from low erucic acid rapeseed oils (0.1–4.8%) demonstrated lesions in male rats (147, 197–200). Minor lesions, not significantly different from those in the control animals, were observed when rats were fed low erucic acid rapeseed oil containing 0.3–1.4% erucic acid (187, 201, 202). After the feeding of one of the oils containing 0.3% erucic acid (187), no lesions were found despite serial-sectioning of the whole heart. On the contrary, all animals fed high erucic acid rapeseed oil, both male and female, were reported to show lesions.

Partial hydrogenation was found to reduce the cardiopathenicity of low erucic acid rapeseed oil but not of high erucic acid rapeseed oil (203). Although many feeding studies on rapeseed oil low in erucic acid have been reported, the varying and sometimes high frequency of similar lesions in control rats makes interpretation difficult.

COMPARATIVE ANIMAL STUDIES

Ducklings

In a study (204) in which young ducklings were fed a rapeseed oil with 8.5% erucic acid as 50% of the energy, the heart was pale after two weeks (fatty infiltration) in five animals out of ten. After three months the hearts of six animals were normal while the other four had enlarged hearts (204).

Pigs

Pigs receiving low erucic acid rapeseed oil did not show any lipidosis, but did show cellular infiltration and fibrosis. These effects were milder than in pigs fed high erucic acid rapeseed oil (204a).

63

A few other studies of the effects of rapeseed oils in pigs have been published. In these studies, infiltration of mononuclear cells was independent of the kind of oil fed; the control animals, not given rapeseed oil, showed such infiltration in from 4% to 67% of the hearts examined.

Monkeys

In a six-month study with cynomolgus monkeys fed low erucic acid rapeseed oil no long-term lipidosis was observed, and also no difference existed between the hearts of those animals and the control animals in respect of the few long-term lesions observed (204b).

BACKGROUND LESIONS IN CARDIAC TISSUE

Lesions in the hearts found after prolonged feeding of rapeseed oils are unspecific. They can be induced by several dietary components as well as other agents and are frequently observed in the control animals not given rapeseed oil. In some experiments the presence of lesions in animals on control diets was reported to be as high as 50%; however, frequencies of about 10–30% were more common. The causes of these lesions were not identified, but they could not be connected to any known dietary components. Undoubtedly, a high frequency of myocardial alterations in the control animals tends to obscure interpretation of the results obtained by testing low erucic acid rapeseed oil.

CAUSES OF LONG-TERM LESIONS

It has been proposed (197) that in addition to erucic acid some other characteristic of rapeseed oil was responsible for the long-term lesions. Possible causes were suggested: the low content of saturated fatty acids, an unbalanced ratio between saturated and monounsaturated fatty acids, or unsaponifiable matter in the oil. Testing of the hypothesis that an unbalanced fatty acid composition was the cause showed that only when erucic acid was incorporated into the mixtures of synthesized fats could long-term lesions be induced in male rats. Other researchers suggested that the long-chain fatty acids (20 carbon atoms or more) were the sole cause. They interpreted the residual lesions induced by low erucic acid rapeseed oil as being caused by the erucic acid still present. However, attempts to concentrate or eliminate a toxic factor were unsuccessful.

CONCLUSIONS

Reports from several laboratories indicate that a short-term dietary intake of brassica oils with a high percentage of erucic acid causes transient diffuse myocardial lipidosis (fat deposition of the myocardium) in several animal species. The accumulation of triglycerides in the heart of the rat reaches a peak after about one week and falls to almost normal levels by four weeks despite continued feeding of the dietary fat. The accumulation of triglycerides in the heart is directly proportional to the amount of erucic acid in the diet.

There has been discussion of the possibility that erucic acid is less efficiently oxidized and therefore accumulates in the form of triglycerides in the heart cells. Experimental data indicate that erucoyl carnitine competitively inhibits the oxidation of other acyl carnitines in the heart mitochondria. The fatty acid compositions of the main membrane phospholipids of rat heart mitochondria — i.e., phosphatidylcholine, phosphatidylethanolamine and cardiolipin — are influenced by dietary erucic acid.

Long-term feeding of high erucic acid brassica oils induces focal necrotic lesions with reactive cellular infiltration leading to fibrotic changes in the rat heart muscle. It has been reported that in the rat erucic acid *per se* is a cardiopathogenic agent and can induce cardiac necrosis and fibrosis.

Studies of low erucic acid brassica oils show that they permit the same growth in the rat as other fats and oils.

In some laboratories long-term feeding of brassica oils low in erucic acid has been reported to increase necrotic lesions in the myocardium above background levels, but the severity was less than that found with high erucic acid rapeseed oil. Partial hydrogenation reduced the cardiopathogenicity of low erucic acid rapeseed oil. Morphological studies of other organs have revealed no deleterious effects from rapeseed oils low in erucic acid (22:1, n–9).

At present there is considerable controversy as to whether the long-term lesions in test animals produced by brassica oils low in erucic acid are due to the erucic acid or to another factor.

Three theories have been proposed.

1. The lesions are the effects of erucic acid still present in the oils.

2. The nontriglyceride part of the oil may contain a cardiopathogenic component.

3. There is an imbalance in the fatty acid composition which is not tolerated by the cardiac tissue.

In view of the present knowledge from animal studies, it seems prudent to recommend for populations in which fat constitutes a high proportion of dietary energy (a) the reduction of the erucic acid in brassica oils and/or (b) the blending or use of brassica oils with other fats and oils. This recommendation, which could be of special importance for children, might have to be modified in the light of further data from human studies.

Table 11. – Production/trade/apparent consumption of marine oils and partially hydrogenated marine oils (PHMO) in selected countries, 1976

| Country | Raw marine oil[1] | | | Long-chain fatty acids in PHMO | | | PHMO per caput per year[3] |
| | Production and/or imports | Export | Apparent consumption[2] | Carbon chain length | | | |
				C-20	C-22	C-22:1	
	Thousand metric tons			Percent			Kilograms
Norway	4 190	150	40	18-24	18-28	10-16	8.2
Denmark	4 75	60	15	18-22	24-28	10-16	2.5
Iceland	4 30	30	0	18-22	24-28	10-16	nil
USSR	4 80	0	80	–	–	–	0.3
United Kingdom	5 190	6 20	170	18	15	13	2.5
Germany, F.R.	5 140	6 20	120	18	12	10	1.6
Netherlands	5 100	6 70	30	18	12	10	2.2
Sweden	5 15	0	15	12-18	8-12	2-6	1.7
Canada	4 10	0	10	18-22	24-32	20-25	0.5
USA	4 100	80	7 20	12-18	8-12	2-6	nil
Peru	4 150	60	90	18-25	10-13	2-6	5.0
South Africa	4 55	15	40	20-25	12-14	3-8	1.5
Japan	4 120	60	60	–	–	–	0.5

[1] The data cover about 80–85% of the total world production and are calculated means for the years 1972-76. The data are compiled from official statistics and from Norwegian industrial statistics. See also *Oil World*, 18:424 (1977). – [2] Including food and nonfood uses. – [3] Assuming that approximately 85% of the raw marine oil is converted to PHMO. – [4] Own production. – [5] Own production and/or import. – [6] Calculated on the assumption that 50% of the fat in bakery products is from PHMO and that the bakery products contain approximately 10% fat. – [7] PHMO is not allowed in foods. The given amount is used for technical purposes.

Health implications of long-chain fatty acids in marine oils

INTRODUCTION

Marine oils have always been part of the human diet, mainly consumed as fresh fish or oils from marine animals. No epidemiological data indicate that the intake of a reasonable quantity of fats of marine origin carries a specific risk factor for human health.

In some countries (Table 11) partially hydrogenated marine oils (PHMO) have been consumed as a component of margarine and shortening for over fifty years. Commercial marine oils are generally divided into two broad classes: anchoveta and menhaden oils, which are low (1–4%) in docosenoic acids (22:1), and oils from herring, capelin, sand launce and some marine mammals, all of which contain noticeably higher quantities (10–20%; *see* Table 12). The principal docosenoic acid is cetoleic acid (22:1, *n*–11). The docosenoic acid content is not greatly altered by partial hydrogenation, but positional and geometric isomers are formed in the product. Generally, the positions of the remaining unsaturated bonds are close to those in the parent structure (*n*–11), and about half of them have a trans configuration. The same observation has been made for the eicosenoic acids (20:1), which are often present in quantities comparable to the docosenoic acids (Table 12).

BIOCHEMISTRY AND NUTRITIONAL VALUE

Various *in vitro* experiments with carnitine esters of different isomers of docosenoic acids (22:1) from PHMO indicate some differences in their metabolism. Brassidoyl carnitine (trans 22:1, *n*–9) inhibits both mitochondrial oxidation of palmitoyl carnitine and respiration less than erucoyl carnitine (22:1, *n*–9) and ceteoleoyl carnitine (22:1, *n*–11). All carnitine esters of docosenoic acids (22:1) seem to be relatively better oxidized in the liver than in the heart mitochondria (195). The mitochondrial metabolism of docosenoic acids is more fully discussed on pages 61 and 62.

Fatty acids present in PHMO are readily assimilated by test animals and do not affect growth provided that there is an adequate supply of dietary essential fatty acids, similar to that found in other edible oils (205).

SHORT- AND LONG-TERM EFFECTS ON THE HEART IN ANIMALS

The result of studies on short- and long-term effects of PHMO on the heart in animals are summarized in Table 13. It is accepted that docosenoic-acid-induced cardiac lipidosis can be demonstrated in experimental animals when PHMO is fed continuously as part of high-fat diets. This

TABLE 12. – FATTY ACID PATTERNS OF PARTIALLY HYDROGENATED MARINE OILS (PHMO) FROM DIFFERENT RAW MATERIALS

Source	PHMO melting point °C	Fatty acid													
		14:0	16:0	16:1	18:0	18:1	18:x[1]	20:0	20:1	20:x[1]	22:0	22:1	22:x[1]
Capelin	30/32	6-9	12-16	6-10	3-5	16-20	2-4	1-3	10-17	5-8	1-3	10-16	2-8
Capelin	38/40	6-9	14-16	6-9	6-8	12-15	1-3	3-5	10-13	3-7	4-6	12-14	2-5
Herring	35/37	7.4	14.9	5.6	6.5	13	2.9	4.8	11.3	5.1	5.3	14.1	5.2
Herring	30/32	8	12-14	8-9	2-3	12-16	2-4	2-4	16-20	2-4	2-3	20-23	3.0
Menhaden	34	9.7	21	14.6	5.7	15.3	2.5	1.0	6.4	12.0	0.5	1.8	6.0
Menhaden	40	9.0	23.2	11.6	9.5	15.9	1.4	3.1	8.5	7.4	1.1	3.4	3.6

[1] Indicates 2–4 double bonds.

TABLE 13. – SUMMARY OF RESULTS FROM VARIOUS LABORATORIES OF THE FEEDING OF HIGH-FAT DIETS, INCLUDING MARINE OILS AND PHMO, TO EXPERIMENTAL ANIMALS

Species	Place of work	Result
Rat	Ottawa (141)	Partially hydrogenated capelin and herring oils gave acute lipidosis [1] above 4–5 energy %. [2] Long-term lesions observed in various studies. Raw anchovy oil gave no lipidosis [1] at 1 energy %. [2]
	Halifax (210)	Partially hydrogenated and raw fish oil of 10 energy % [2] gave lesions comparable to control oil after 16 weeks.
	Dijon (211, 212)	Partially hydrogenated herring oil gave acute lipidosis [1] at 9 energy %. [2] Fewer lesions on partially hydrogenated herring oil than on rapeseed oil at a similar docosenoic (22:1) acid level after 16 weeks.
	Oslo (213)	Partially hydrogenated capelin oil gave an increasing incidence of acute lipidosis [1] above 2 energy %; [2] after 16 weeks long-term lesions were comparable to those from control oil.
	Bergen (205)	Partially hydrogenated capelin oil at 6 energy % [2] and raw capelin oil at 4 energy % gave no lipidosis.
Pig	Oslo (214)	Partially hydrogenated and raw capelin oils at 7 energy % [2] gave no acute lipidosis. [1] Mild lipidosis developed eventually. No lesions above control oil number after 1 year.
Primate	Saskatoon (215)	Partially hydrogenated herring oil at 12 energy % [2] gave lipidosis [1] comparable to control diet after 6 and 12 months, but no important lesions during those periods.

[1] Lipidosis detection either chemical (gravimetric determination of lipid, triglyceride or fatty acid) or histopathological (oil-red-0 staining and microscopic evaluation). – [2] Percent of dietary energy contributed by docosenoic acid (22:1).

effect is most marked when the oil belongs to the high docosenoic acid group (Table 12), contributing more than 4–6% of the energy from these acids to the diet, and seems directly related to the content of docosenoic acids in the diet. In the rat the disappearance of lipidosis on continued feeding (adaptation) parallels that observed for brassica oils. The appearance of long-term lesions, discussed above, shows species differences (Table 13). The lesions often do not, however, differ in number and severity from those observed in control groups. There appear to be important differences in the responses of different species in both short-

and long-term effects. No data on pathological changes in other organs have yet been reported.

POSSIBLE EFFECTS ON THE HUMAN HEART

Because differences exist in the degree of myocardial lipidosis among species, and because the mechanism of adaptation to docosenoic acid likewise appears to vary in many respects among them, great care should be taken in extrapolating to man the observations of lipidosis phenomena in animals. However, in view of the fact that myocardial lipidosis can be induced in the non-human primate, it is not unlikely that the same phenomena may be observed in man on a high-fat diet rich in docosenoic acid.

If lipidosis due to intake of docosenoic acid does occur in man, it would probably have been noted by pathologists in countries where the consumption of docosenoic acids from either marine or vegetable sources is relatively high.

Recent surveys and epidemiological studies indicate that cardiovascular diseases are uncommon in Eskimo populations in Greenland which have had a lifetime exposure to natural marine oils containing docosenoic acid (207, 208).

In a study of fatty changes in 34 Finnish subjects over 20 years of age who had died suddenly from mechanical trauma or rapid suffocation, parenchymal fatty changes assessed as medium or profuse were found in about 50% of the cases (206). This suggests that the lipidosis phenomenon, at least in a mild form, may be relatively common among this population, which is not generally exposed to large quantities of docosenoic acid of any origin.

The hearts of 54 Norwegian men aged 20–69 who had died suddenly in accidents were screened from some 600 hearts as being free of myocardial infarction, coronary thrombosis, myocardial hypertrophy and valvular diseases.[1] Histochemical lipidosis, mostly moderate in degree, was found in 60% of the hearts. The fatty acids of the total lipids in the 54 hearts were found to contain docosenoic acid (22:1) at 1% or less of the fatty acids. Canadian data from a more limited study of the fatty acids from human heart triglycerides also showed less than 1% docosenoic acid (22:1).[2]

These forensic data show that very mild cardiac lipidosis, not necessarily associated with deposits of docosenoic acid, may be widespread in humans consuming a Western high-fat diet irrespective of the type of fat consumed. Published studies indicate that diffuse myocarditis in

---

[1] H. Svaar (in press). – [2] R.G. Ackman (in press).

70

man is not unusual, but no report associates this condition with high-fat intake in general or with docosenoic acid originating from PHMO in particular (209). In the examination of the 54 human hearts reported above, no evidence of multifocal heart muscle lesions of the type seen in rats fed rapeseed oil was found in normal men from a population suspected of long-term exposure to PHMO.

In many feeding experiments on rats there was a considerable time lag between the appearance of lipidosis and the finding of muscle cell necrosis, suggesting that moderate lipidosis *per se* is not injurious to the heart muscle cell. The absence of acute heart muscle cell necrosis or myocardial fibrosis, in a human population exposed to PHMO, despite the concurrent presence of mild to moderate cardiac lipidosis, supports this view.

CONCLUSIONS

1. Cardiac lipidosis can be induced in certain experimental animals by continuous feeding of PHMO containing high proportions of docosenoic acids (22:1) in a high-fat diet. The increase of cardiac lipidosis above control levels is related to the dietary concentration of docosenoic acid. Although the effects of PHMO are qualitatively similar to those of rapeseed oils containing erucic acid (22:1, *n*–9), quantitatively the effects of PHMO are somewhat milder.

2. On the available evidence relating to PHMO there is no support for a relationship between lipidosis observed in experimental animals and the long-term myocardial lesions sometimes observed in the same animal experiments.

3. Mild lipidosis without long-term myocardial lesions was found in a number of hearts from human populations on high-fat diets. As only two populations, one suspected of exposure to PHMO and one not, have been examined critically, additional studies are urgently required.

4. No harmful effect in man has been attributed to the intake of unprocessed marine lipids.

5. In the light of present knowledge from animal studies it seems prudent to recommend for populations in which fat constitutes a high proportion of dietary energy the blending or the direct use of partially hydrogenated marine oils (PHMO) with other fats and oils. This recommendation, which may be of special importance for children, may need to be modified in the light of further data from human studies.

Biological significance of uneven fatty acids

Fatty acids of uneven carbon numbers are at present minor constituents of the human diet. There is, however, a possibility of consuming increased amounts of them from preparations of single-cell proteins grown on n-alkanes. Metabolically, uneven fatty acids are degraded by beta-oxidation to yield acetic and propionic acids which are utilized normally. Polyunsaturated uneven fatty acids may have essential fatty acid activity if the cis double bonds are methylene-interrupted, normally in the same position as in the next higher homologue (216).

Although most biosynthetic uneven fatty acids have 15 and 17 carbon chain lengths, much of the published work in this field has dealt with the 11 carbon chain length, the glucogenic property of which was found to assist in the maintenance of serum glucose and liver glycogen during starvation.

Lipids of single-cell protein preparations containing a high concentration of uneven fatty acids are incorporated into tissue lipids, but have not been shown to affect functional capacity (217). This indicates that the level of consumption of lipids in single-cell protein preparations appears to be within the metabolic capability of mammals. This conclusion accords with that of the Protein-Calorie Advisory Group (218).

9. RECENT TRENDS IN PRODUCTION, TRADE AND CONSUMPTION OF FATS AND OILS

Production and trade

The production of visible fats and oils is summarized in Table 14. Of the total production, about 70% is of vegetable and 30% of animal origin. About three quarters of the total output is used for human food, and the remainder for such products as detergents, soaps, paints and animal feeds. Many fats and oils are joint products (e.g., meat/animal fats, oilseeds/oilmeals). The supply of fats and oils is therefore linked not only to the demand for them but also to the demand for their joint products.

World output and consumption of fats and oils have been increasing by nearly 1.2 million metric tons a year over the last decade. The most important increases in output have taken place in soybean, palm, rapeseed and sunflowerseed oils. Developing countries, in spite of their need for increased domestic consumption and more export, have only just maintained their share of total output.

Annual net exports currently amount to about 10 million metric tons, equally divided between the developed and the developing plus centrally planned countries. They originate from a large number of developing countries and relatively few developed countries (principally the United States, which is by far the largest exporter of fats and oils). The share of developing countries in exports (but not in production) fell late in the 1960s owing to a relatively slow growth in output and rapidly increasing domestic consumption (Table 15). In recent years, however, the exports of a few — notably Malaysia, Brazil, Indonesia and Ivory Coast — have begun to increase. On the other hand, in other developing countries the volume of exports has declined or shown only marginal growth.

While the largest importers continue to be Western Europe and Japan, imports into developing countries have been growing at a faster rate (over 7% a year) and now account for about one quarter of the world total (Table 16).

Importing developing countries are widely spread over the different regions. In Africa, the Mahgreb countries are the most important; in the Near East, Egypt, Iran and Iraq; in Latin America, Cuba, Mexico, Venezuela, Brazil, Peru, Chile and Colombia; and in Asia, India, Pakistan,

TABLE 14. – PRODUCTION OF VISIBLE OILS AND FATS
(Thousand metric tons)

Commodity	1964-66 average				1969-71 average				1973-75 average			
	World	Developed countries	Developing countries	C.P.C.[1]	World	Developed countries	Developing countries	C.P.C.[1]	World	Developed countries	Developing countries	C.P.C.[1]
Soybean oil	4 530	3 500	70	960	6 530	5 220	310	1 000	8 760	6 280	1 420	1 060
Sunflowerseed oil	2 740	140	260	2 340	3 760	240	420	3 100	4 050	470	470	3 110
Groundnut oil	3 300	160	2 770	370	3 410	220	2 780	410	3 110	240	2 440	430
Cottonseed oil	2 540	960	940	640	2 530	690	1 100	740	2 990	800	1 250	940
Palm oil	1 400	–	1 350	50	1 860	–	1 750	110	2 730	–	2 580	150
Coconut oil	2 370	–	2 350	20	2 430	–	2 410	20	2 550	–	2 530	20
Rapeseed oil	1 580	390	560	630	2 050	720	730	600	2 550	930	820	800
Olive oil	1 300	1 030	260	10	1 340	1 070	260	10	1 440	1 080	350	10
Palm-kernel oil	550	–	540	10	590	–	580	10	650	–	630	20
Others	1 440	480	760	200	1 620	500	930	190	1 810	610	1 000	200
Total vegetable oils	21 750	6 660	9 860	5 230	26 120	8 660	11 270	6 190	30 640	10 410	13 490	6 740
Total animal & marine fats and oils	13 430	8 490	1 680	3 260	14 490	8 920	1 990	3 580	15 230	8 920	1 980	4 330
Total edible fats and oils	35 180	15 150	11 540	8 490	40 610	17 580	13 260	9 770	45 870	19 330	15 470	11 070
PERCENT	100	43	33	24	100	43	33	24	100	42	34	24

[1] C.P.C. = Centrally planned countries.

TABLE 15. – NET EXPORTS OF OILS AND FATS [1]
(Thousand metric tons)

	1964–66 average	1969–71 average	1973–75 average
Developed	3 460	4 460	4 940
Developing	3 630	3 550	4 370
Centrally planned	390	910	540
WORLD TOTAL	7 480	8 920	9 850

[1] Aggregated export supplies (i.e., gross exports minus gross imports) of net exporting countries. Trade figures include the equivalent of oilseeds traded.

Bangladesh and the Republic of Korea. In addition to these, there are ten other countries whose imports of fats and oils averaged over 30 000 metric tons a year in 1972–74. In recent years food aid shipments have provided about 10% of the requirements of developing countries, divided more or less equally between gifts and concessional sales.

Consumption

In addition to the visible (separated) fats and oils of plant and animal origin dealt with in the preceding chapters, there are the invisible (unseparated) oils and fats deriving from other food groups: grains, nuts and seeds, fruits and vegetables, meats, dairy products, eggs and fish. As shown in Table 17, invisible fats are more abundant in the diet than visible ones and in most regions amount to 60% of the total fat supply.

In the developed countries the total per caput supply [1] of fats available for human consumption in 1974 was 126 g (1 134 kcal; 4.7 MJ) a day, of which 86 g (775 kcal; 3.2 MJ), or 70%, were of animal origin. The supply of fats of animal origin in almost all regions of the developed countries is twice as great as that of plant origin. In the developing countries the total fat supply is much lower, amounting to only 35 g (315 kcal; 1.3 MJ) a day, of which only 14 g (126 kcal; 0.53 MJ), or 40%, were of animal origin. Among the developing countries, only in Latin America and in the Asian countries with centrally planned economies

[1] The data refer not to the quantity of fat actually ingested (actual consumption data are not available) but to the supply available for human consumption at kitchen level as estimated from data on production, trade, stocks and nonfood uses.

TABLE 16. – NET IMPORTS OF OILS AND FATS [1]

	1964–66 average	1969–71 average	1973–75 average
Developed	5 820	6 540	6 670
Developing	1 420	1 980	2 550
Centrally planned	450	440	420
WORLD TOTAL	7 690	8 960	9 640

[1] Aggregated import requirements (i.e., gross imports less exports) of net importing countries. Trade figures include the oil equivalent of oilseeds traded.

are the supplies of animal fats of the same magnitude as those derived from plants. Africa and especially the Far East have the lowest supplies of animal fats. The low levels prevailing in these regions are attributable primarily to the low availability of animal products, in particular, meat and dairy products; there the average per caput consumption of both visible and invisible fats and oils of animal origin does not exceed 8 g (72 kcal; 0.3 MJ) a day. Among the developed countries, Japan is notable for its relatively low supply of fats and oils of animal origin.

For the world as a whole, the energy supplied by fat averages nearly 22% of all energy supplied by food. The proportion of energy derived from fat is 33% for developed countries and over 40% for the high-income countries of America and Europe. By contrast, in the developing countries fats supply on average only 14% of the dietary energy.

Inequalities in fat consumption are to an extent explained by the ecological environment, which determines the consumption pattern. This is particularly true for populations living in a subsistence economy. In monetary economies, household income appears to be the main variable explaining changes in fat consumption. Thus, the developed market economy countries, Eastern Europe and the USSR in 1974 utilized 61% of the visible fats and oils and 59% of the total fat available for human consumption, although they had only 28% of the world's population.

Figure 5 illustrates the changes in per caput supply of total fat in relation to changes in per caput income during the period 1965–74.

In the developing countries, which consume small amounts of fats and oils, the elasticity of demand is very great, but rapidly increasing populations and slow income growth have severely limited any improvement in per caput consumption. This is particularly evident in the African and Asian regions. Accordingly, the gaps in per caput consumption

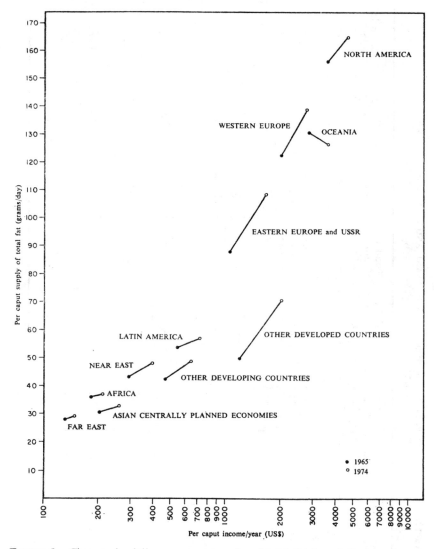

FIGURE 5. Changes in daily per caput supply of total fat in relation to changes in per caput income, by regions, 1965–74.

between developed and developing countries in 1965 widened for both visible fats and oils and total fats in 1974. Therefore, in virtually all developing countries, the potential for increased per caput consumption is enormous, although its realization will depend on higher incomes unless other measures to increase availability at low prices are instituted.

77

TABLE 17. — SUPPLY OF INVISIBLE AND VISIBLE FATS OF PLANT AND ANIMAL ORIGIN, 1974
(Grams per caput a day)

	Visible fats and oils	Invisible fats and oils	Total fat of plant origin	Total fat of animal origin	Total fat	Total calorie supply	Fat/calorie ratio [1]
Developed market economies .	58.7	75.7	44.9	89.5	134.4	3 333	36.3
North America	65.1	100.0	45.2	119.9	165.1	3 492	42.5
Western Europe	65.8	73.0	49.0	89.8	138.9	3 411	36.6
Oceania	42.1	85.6	24.7	103.0	127.7	3 355	34.3
Others	30.5	40.6	36.3	34.8	71.1	2 851	22.4
Eastern Europe & USSR ..	42.7	66.4	30.8	78.3	109.0	3 511	27.9
All developed countries	53.5	72.6	40.3	85.8	126.2	3 391	33.5
Developing market economies	15.9	20.7	24.3	12.3	36.7	2 197	15.0
Africa	15.6	20.9	28.3	8.2	36.5	2 118	15.5
Latin America	24.7	32.3	28.7	28.3	56.9	2 555	20.0
Near East	24.2	24.2	31.2	17.2	48.4	2 464	17.7
Far East	12.0	16.8	20.8	8.0	28.8	2 068	12.5
Others	14.6	35.0	25.9	23.7	49.6	2 329	19.2
Asian centrally planned economies	8.5	24.5	16.0	17.0	33.0	2 331	12.7
All developing countries	13.6	21.9	21.7	13.8	35.5	2 239	14.3
World	24.9	36.5	27.0	34.4	61.4	2 567	21.5

[1] Percent calories provided by total fat as percent of total calorie supply.

TABLE 18.

TABLE 18. – CHANGES IN THE SUPPLY OF VISIBLE AND INVISIBLE FATS
BETWEEN 1965 AND 1974
(Grams per caput a day)

	Developed countries		Developing countries		World	
	1965	1974	1965	1974	1965	1974
Visible fat						
Plant	25.1	30.5	9.6	10.7	14.4	16.3
Animal	22.3	23.0	2.7	2.9	8.8	8.6
Invisible fat						
Plant	9.7	9.8	11.1	11.0	10.7	10.7
Animal	53.0	62.8	10.6	10.9	23.8	25.8
Total fat	110.1	126.1	34.0	35.5	57.7	61.4

By contrast, in the developed countries the intake of fats increased over the decade, most notably owing to a considerable rise in household income. This is particularly marked for Japan, the Eastern European countries and the Mediterranean countries of Western Europe, which in terms of consumption were in a medium position in 1965. Several high-income countries have reached or are reaching a saturation threshold for some visible fats and oils. Thus, income elasticities of demand for butter are close to zero in the European Common Market countries and are even negative in Canada, the USA, the Scandinavian countries, Australia and New Zealand.

In Western Europe and North America the increase in intake of total fats has been more moderate than the rise in household income would lead one to assume; in Oceania intake has declined.

These changes are the result of several trends. In Oceania, the only region showing an overall decline in fat consumption, the increase in the supply of vegetable fats was more than offset by a decline in the supply of fats of animal origin.

For the developed countries as a whole, during the period 1965–74 the supply of visible fats of plant origin available for human consumption increased by about 5 g per caput a day, and at the same time invisible fats of animal origin showed a notable increase of 10 g per caput a day.

For the developing countries as a whole, the changes were minor, mainly increases in visible fats and oils of plant origin, as shown in Table 18. The supply of animal fats changed very little.

79

10. IMPACT OF PLANT AND ANIMAL BREEDING AND MANAGEMENT ON QUALITY AND COMPOSITION OF FATS AND OILS

Plant breeding

To meet greatly increased demands for all forms of fats, including edible vegetable oils, developed countries — in addition to increasing their own production — have also sought to overcome certain natural limitations in the oils by genetic manipulation. On the other hand, the prime aim in developing countries has been to increase supplies of conventional oils through expansion of both cultivated areas and yields per unit area.

ALTERATION OF OIL COMPOSITION

Work in Canada and Sweden has resulted in the breeding of strains of rapeseed that yield an oil almost free (below 0.5%) of erucic acid (22:1, n–9), which in traditional strains had been about 40%. The α-linolenic acid (18:3, n–3) content is elevated in the low erucic acid strains, but is associated with flavour and rancidity problems.

These new varieties comprise a substantial part of the rapeseed crop in several countries (e.g., Canada and Sweden). The fatty acid composition of these oils as percentages of total oil is as follows:

palmitic acid (16:0)	3
stearic acid (18:0)	2
oleic acid (18:1, n–9)	50–65
linoleic acid (18:2, n–6)	20
α-linolenic acid (18:3, n–3) ...	10
eicosenoic acid (20:1, n–9)	0–10
erucic acid (22:1, n–9)	0–5

Apart from the change in fatty acid composition, it has been possible through plant breeding to reduce appreciably the content of glucosinolates.

A major problem with cottonseed oil has been the presence of the pigment gossypol, which is toxic to nonruminants, including man. Selective breeding has eliminated gossypol glands from the seeds but has rendered the cotton boll itself more susceptible to insect attack. From the normal linoleic-rich varieties, selective breeding of safflower has yielded an oil rich in oleic acid (18:1, n–9).

Breeding programmes are slow and very expensive, even when rapid techniques such as irradiation and aseptic cell cultures are used. The possibility that irradiation mutants may revert to type must also be borne in mind. Such breeding programmes should be embarked upon only if there is an exceptionally sound reason.

IMPROVING OIL YIELD

There are several approaches to breeding for improvement in oil yield. One is to develop varieties having a larger density or a greater proportion of oil in the oil-bearing seed, fruit or nut. Other approaches include reduction of hull content, as has been done with the sunflower and the safflower, or reduction or elimination of shattering, a course being pursued with sesame. Oil production can also be increased by developing early-maturing varieties and those requiring less moisture. Improved analytical screening methods are available to assist the breeder, such as the rapid determination of oil content by nondestructive nuclear magnetic resonance, rapid gas-liquid chromatography techniques for fatty acid analysis and fast protein estimation by dye binding techniques. In practice, a higher oil content in an oilseed is frequently accompanied by a higher protein content.

CONCLUSIONS

Since oil palm yields several times more oil per unit area than many other oilseed crops, and since soybean has received widespread publicity, some developing countries could be unduly induced to grow these crops. Palm oil contains a high proportion of saturated fatty acids and a low proportion of essential fatty acids. The soybean has a relatively low oil content, and the bulk of the produce is a protein oilcake that may not always have high economic value within developing countries. The higher yields of newly introduced varieties frequently result simply from the attention given to fertilization and irrigation, which if similarly applied to traditional crops might yield just as satisfactory results. Therefore, a good general principle would be to plan for maximum possible oilseed diversity, both to stabilize yields and protect overall world supplies against gluts of individual oils.

Knowledge of biosynthetic pathways of triglyceride synthesis would greatly assist breeding efforts. In attempting genetic manipulation the levels of minor components of oilseed lipids such as phospholipids, tocopherols and other lipid associates should also be routinely checked, as these would be relevant to human nutrition. When a new oilseed has proved its potential and is ready to be raised on a large scale, suitable systems of management and marketing must be developed. Continued efforts should be made to explore and develop other natural oil-bearing plants not yet in cultivation.

In considering other crops, however, green vegetables, although they have a low fat content, should not be overlooked; they are a source of α-linolenic acid (18:3, *n*–3) and provide important amounts of carotenoids (pro-vitamin A), vitamin E and other vitamins and minerals.

Animal breeding and management

CARCASS AND TISSUE FATS

The intake of foods of animal origin tends to increase with affluence. In developing countries poultry products and, in certain societies, other small animals are important contributors of foods of animal origin. Poultry meat has a low content of saturated fats and is a good source of long-chain essential fatty acid (EFA). In developed countries, pork and beef are important animal foods. Increasing animal food intake could have three general consequences for human nutrition: (*i*) intensive animal production systems tend to yield foods high in fats; (*ii*) the proportion of dietary saturated fatty acids rises; and (*iii*) cholesterol intake tends to increase.

The principal components of fats in animal tissues and milk are triglycerides, fatty acids, cholesterol and phospholipids. The triglycerides are the predominant lipids of adipose tissue and of milk. Although cow's milk has relatively low amounts of EFA (about 1 energy %), it is nonetheless an important source of energy and essential nutrients.

Fats in meat, liver, kidneys and other offal are naturally rich in long-chain EFA as a component of their structural phospholipids. Under intensive management systems, increased adipose fat deposition conceals this characteristic. This fat consists mainly of triglycerides rich in saturated fatty acids (219, 220).

In nonruminants the fatty acid composition of the adipose fat reflects the nature of the dietary fat. In ruminants biohydrogenation in the rumen raises the content of saturated acids and lowers that of EFA both in adipose and milk fat. Cholesterol occurs either free or esterified to a fatty acid, generally unsaturated. Its concentration is greatest in cells with a high degree of membrane development (e.g., brain, liver, kidney).

QUANTITATIVE ASPECTS

During animal growth there is a physiological stage at which the fattening phase begins (222); prior to this, protein is deposited proportionately to fat deposition. The onset of this phase varies with species and sex. This stage is reached sooner in early maturing animals, and at a given weight they are therefore preferable to other types. By selection of suitable genotypes it is possible to obtain carcasses of various weights while maintaining the juvenile characteristics of low adipose fat and high protein content.

The system of production management also significantly affects the shape of the growth curve for a given type of animal (222). The energy/protein ratio of the diet and the activity patterns of the animals are generally varied to modify fat deposition (223). This does not apply to wild herbivores nor to domesticated herbivores on rangelands. Wild herbivores deposit little adipose fat and have a carcass that is high in protein (224). Ruminants finished in the feedlot are often fed for maximum growth regardless of size, and very fat animals sometimes result.

Intensively reared animals with high-fat carcasses of the order of 30% may provide more fat than other nutrients (220). This fat is expensive in terms of efficiency of feed conversion, and its production loses sight of the true nutritional value of the animal product, which lies in muscle tissue and offal.

QUALITATIVE ASPECTS

The adipose fats of wild herbivores and birds are generally more polyunsaturated than those of their domestic counterparts (219, 225, 225a). It is therefore technically possible to modify animal fat with dietary fats, as has long been recognized by producers of poultry and pig meats. Thus the fatty acid composition of fats of animal origin can be modified and the cholesterol content of pork products can be reduced by increasing the dietary polyunsaturated fatty acids (221).

In ruminants it has been shown that protected lipid supplements can bypass the rumen biohydrogenation process (226). At the same time, proteins are protected from proteolysis and digested normally in the small intestine. Oils or fats emulsified in protein solutions can be protected from ruminal lipolysis and hydrogenation by formaldehyde treatment of the emulsion. When such protected polyunsaturated oils are fed to cattle and sheep, the concentration of linoleic (18:2, n–6) and α-linolenic (18:3, n–3) acids both in tissue fats and in milk fats is increased. The nonfunctional rumens in veal and lamb make their fats susceptible to dietary modification (227). Milk fat is dependent on breed of cow, stage of lactation and feed. The linoleic acid content of milk fat can be raised to a level of 20% of the fatty acids by feeding encapsulated fats; the increased transfer of such fats into milk can also raise both milk fat concentrations and total daily secretion.

Products with an elevated linoleic acid content are more susceptible to oxidative deterioration. Their flavour has been found to be little changed in beef and veal, but may be of concern in sheep meats for some consumers.

CONCLUSIONS

Foods of animal and plant origin complement each other in terms of agriculture production and human nutrition. However, in aiming for a balanced diet, competition with human food production should be avoided whenever alternative animal production systems are available — hence the importance of using agricultural industrial by-products for animal feeding in developing countries. Alternative feeding schemes for poultry, pig and beef are already available in those countries.

More attention should be paid to the fact that although animal tissues are naturally rich in long-chain EFA, intensive fattening destroys this property. The most economical way to solve this problem would seem to be a control or reduction of fattening with a consequent saving of high energy foods.

The nutritional characteristics of poultry products, offals and wildlife resources, which may be major sources of animal foods in developing countries, should be given more attention in the future.

11. RECOMMENDATIONS

A number of recommendations arose from discussion of the papers presented at the Joint FAO/WHO Expert Consultation on the Role of Dietary Fats and Oils in Human Nutrition. They basically concern diet, processing and production, on the one hand, and future lines of research, on the other. They are listed below without necessarily implying any order of priority.

General

DIET

1. For population groups with a low energy intake every effort should be made to increase the fat content of the diet so as to raise the energy density of the diet and satisfy energy needs.

2. The recommended minimum energy content of essential fatty acids (EFAs) in the human diet is 3%. Because EFA requirements are higher in pregnancy and lactation, this energy value is raised to 4.5% in pregnancy and 5–7% in lactation (see pages 33–35).

3. Breast-milk substitutes for infants should ideally match the EFA content of human milk; thus weaning diets should contain at least 3% energy as EFA.

4. For population groups with a high incidence of atherosclerosis, obesity and maturity-onset diabetes, the recommended composition of a diet adequate to maintain ideal body weight is 10–15 energy % protein and 30–35 energy % fat. The latter should have a reduced saturated fatty acid content and a linoleic acid (18:2, n–6) content amounting to at least one third of the total fatty acids. The diet should have a low sugar and alcohol content and contain less than 300 mg cholesterol a day.

5. In the light of the present knowledge from animal studies, it seems prudent to recommend for populations in which fat constitutes a high proportion of dietary energy and includes brassica oils that

(a) the levels of erucic acid (22:1, *n*–9) be reduced in brassica oils and/or

(b) brassica oils be blended or mixed with other oils.

This recommendation, which may be of special importance for children, may need to be modified as a result of further data from human studies.

6. In the light of the present knowledge from animal studies, it seems prudent to recommend for populations in which fat constitutes a high proportion of dietary energy and includes partially hydrogenated marine oils that partially hydrogenated marine oils be blended or mixed with other oils. This recommendation, which may be of special importance for children, may also have to be modified as a result of further data from human studies.

7. It is recommended that food products contributing significantly to total fat intake be labelled to indicate the content of total fat and percentages of saturated, cis-monounsaturated, trans-polyunsaturated and all cis-polyunsaturated fatty acids in the fat. Cholesterol should be shown as mg/100 g of the product.

PROCESSING

1. Loss of EFA during hydrogenation and other processes should be minimized.

2. Specific nutrients such as tocopherols and carotenes, if removed in nutritionally significant amounts during refining, should be replaced whenever feasible.

3. Prolonged exposure of polyunsaturated fats to high temperature during refining should be discouraged.

PRODUCTION

1. Edible oil production in developing countries should be increased. Whether achieved by increasing existing edible oil crops or by introducing new varieties, full account should be taken of the need to maintain EFA levels in order to meet the minimum dietary requirements of the nutrient of particular population groups.

2. Excess accumulation of adipose tissue containing highly saturated glycerides should be reduced by changing intensive animal feeding practices or by breeding.

Future lines of research

1. Requirements for the different EFAs — linoleic acid (18:2, *n*–6), α-linolenic acid (18:3, *n*–3) and their long-chain derivatives — with respect to organ development and function.

2. Proportion of EFA utilizable for growth, tissue repair and prostaglandin biosynthesis.

3. Improvement in methods of assessing the EFA status in humans in order to evaluate this condition more accurately.

4. Determination of (*i*) optimum EFA intake during pregnancy, lactation and early development, and (*ii*) the effect of maternal nutrition on lactation, especially milk lipid composition and its effect on child growth and development.

5. Role of EFA in conditions leading to retardation in foetal and child growth and development, especially in protein-energy malnutrition and during nutritional rehabilitation.

6. Effects of early supplementary feeding of high-fat diets adequate in essential fatty acids in two conditions: (*i*) infants breast-fed by malnourished mothers, and (*ii*) early-weaned infants.

7. Blood lipid responses in children to changes of dietary fatty acid composition and the value of the low-saturated fatty acid/high linoleic acid diets for the early prevention of atherosclerosis.

8. Biochemical and physiological mechanisms involved in the effects of dietary fats on blood lipoprotein levels, especially of high-density lipoprotein.

9. Effect of low and high EFA diets on the insulin requirement for the control of diabetes mellitus.

10. Continued evaluation by epidemiological and clinical studies of the possible long-term health effects in subjects consuming diets with relatively high amounts of polyunsaturated fatty acids, trans fatty acids and fatty acids with carbon chain lengths of 20 or more.

11. Vitamin E status in different population groups, especially in those with a low fat intake.

12. Use of improved analytical methods to provide more complete information on the vitamin E content of foods.

13. Effects of dietary antioxidants on EFA metabolism.

14. Extensive investigations into the nature and nutritional effects of by-products developed during fat frying.

15. Examination of all components of brassica oils in an attempt to identify substances other than erucic acid (22:1, n–9) leading to focal necrosis in the hearts of experimental animals.

16. Relationships between consumption of the monounsaturated fatty acids of 20, 22 and 24 carbon chain lengths and their effect on the pathophysiology of the heart and other organs in both the presence and the absence of factors such as hypoxia, stress and alcohol.

17. Differences in metabolism of saturated and monounsaturated fatty acids of 20 and longer carbon chain length and fatty acids of shorter chain length (including clarification of the processes leading to the decrease in lipidosis while the causative agent is still being fed).

18. Determination of the fatty acid composition, including the cis/trans distribution, of foods using modern analytical methods in order to improve the available food composition tables.

19. Further investigation of the biochemical and nutritional properties of the uneven carbon chain length (e.g., 15 and 17) and branched chain fatty acids from single-cell protein preparations intended for human consumption.

Appendix 1

Fatty acid content of some foods

Foods	Fat	Saturated fatty acids			Unsaturated fatty acids				Unsaponifiable matter (g/100 g fat)	Iodine value of fat
		Total	Palmitic	Stearic	Total	Oleic	Linoleic	Other [1]		
Animal products										
MEATS										
Beef	25.1	10.4	6.6	2.7	13.3	10.2	0.6	2.5		47
Mutton	14.8	5.8	2.9	2.2	8.4	6.5	1.0	0.9		40
Pork	35.0	11.4	7.6	3.0	21.9	16.2	3.8	1.9		67
MILK										
Buffalo milk	8.7	5.4	2.5	1.3	2.9	2.3	0.1	0.5	0.3	30
Cow milk	3.5	2.2	0.9	0.4	1.1	0.9	0.1	0.1	0.5	33
Goat milk	3.8	2.4	1.0	0.3	1.3	1.0	0.2	0.1	0.4	37
Human milk	3.2	1.5	1.1	0.2	1.5	1.0	0.3	0.2	0.3	
POULTRY AND EGGS										
Chicken	15.1	6.0	3.7	1.4	8.7	6.4	1.8	0.5		92
Turkey	20.2	5.9	4.4	1.2	13.3	8.7	4.2	0.4		84
Hen egg	11.3	3.4	2.5	0.9	6.0	4.2	1.3	0.5	3.0	84
FISH										
Catfish (fillet)	3.6	0.9	0.6	0.2	2.3	1.0	0.2	1.1		
Herring (whole)	16.4	2.9	1.9	0.2	12.6	2.3	0.2	10.1		
Mackerel (fillet)	12.6	3.2	2.1	0.5	7.6	2.1	0.2	5.3		
Red salmon (fillet) .	8.9	1.4	0.9	0.2	6.9	1.0	0.8	5.1		
Tuna	8.0	2.2	1.6	0.3	5.2	1.4	0.2	3.6		

Composition of foods (g/100 g edible portion)

[1] Includes α-linolenic acid (18:3, n-3) and long-chain essential fatty acids.

Appendix 1

Fatty acid content of some foods (*continued*)

Foods	Fat	Composition of foods (g/100 g edible portion)							Unsaponifiable matter (g/100 g fat)	Iodine value of fat
		Saturated fatty acids			Unsaturated fatty acids					
		Total	Palmitic	Stearic	Total	Oleic	Linoleic	Other [1]		
Animal products										
SEPARATED FATS AND OILS										
Butter	80.1	49.8	21.1	9.7	26.1	20.1	1.8	4.2	0.5	33
Lard	100.0	39.6	23.7	13.0	56.1	40.9	10.0	5.2	0.3	61
Tallow	100.0	48.2	24.8	18.7	46.5	36.0	3.7	6.8	2.5	39
Plant products										
CEREALS AND GRAINS										
Maize (corn)	4.1	0.5	0.4	0.1	3.1	0.9	2.1	0.1	1.6	123
Oats	7.4	1.4	1.2	0.1	5.7	2.6	2.9	0.2		
Rice	2.3	0.6	0.5	trace	1.4	0.5	0.8	0.1	5.0	100
Wheat	2.7	0.4	0.4	trace	1.6	0.3	1.2	0.1	6.0	120
NUTS AND SEEDS										
Brazil-nut	68.2	17.4	10.2	7.1	47.9	22.2	25.4	0.3	0.5	97
Cashew-nut	45.6	9.2	4.3	3.1	33.9	26.2	7.3	0.4	0.5	82
Coconut, mature kernel ...	35.5	31.2	3.0	1.1	2.8	2.0	0.7	0.1	0.2	9
Hazel, filbert-nut ...	64.7	4.6	3.2	1.1	56.7	49.8	6.6	0.3	0.5	86
Groundnut	49.7	9.4	5.3	1.3	37.8	22.9	14.4	0.5	0.7	91
Pilinut	63.0	24.8	17.5	7.3	35.5	29.5	6.0	0.0	0.5	57
Sesame	52.8	8.0	5.0	2.5	42.5	20.6	21.1	0.8	1.0	104

[1] Includes α-linolenic acid (18:3, *n*–3) and long-chain essential fatty acids.

Appendix 1

Fatty acid content of some foods (*concluded*)

Foods	Fat	Composition of foods (g/100 g edible portion)							Unsaponifiable matter (g/100 g fat)	Iodine value of fat
		Saturated fatty acids			Unsaturated fatty acids					
		Total	Palmitic	Stearic	Total	Oleic	Linoleic	Other [1]		
Plant products										
Soybean	17.7	2.7	1.9	0.7	14.3	4.0	9.0	1.3	1.2	133
Walnut	63.4	6.9	4.5	1.3	51.7	9.7	34.9	7.1	0.8	141
SEPARATED FATS AND OILS										
Coconut oil	100.0	87.9	8.4	3.0	8.0	5.7	1.9	0.4	0.2	9
Maize (corn) oil ...	100.0	12.7	10.7	1.7	83.0	24.6	57.4	1.0	1.6	123
Cottonseed oil	100.0	26.1	22.0	2.2	69.6	18.1	50.3	1.2	0.9	112
Mustardseed oil	100.0	5.1	3.0	1.1	86.7	15.8	14.6	[2] 56.3	1.0	119
Olive oil	100.0	14.2	11.5	2.3	81.4	71.5	8.2	1.7	0.8	85
Palm oil	100.0	47.9	42.0	4.3	47.7	37.9	9.0	0.8	1.0	56
Palm-kernel oil	100.0	79.8	7.4	1.9	14.8	13.5	1.1	0.2	0.4	17
Groundnut oil	100.0	19.1	10.7	2.7	76.0	46.0	28.9	1.1	0.7	91
RAPESEED OIL										
High erucic acid ...	100.0	4.3	2.5	0.9	88.4	11.2	12.8	[3] 64.4	0.9	101
Zero erucic acid ...	100.0	6.8	4.8	1.5	88.1	53.2	22.2	[4] 12.7	–	107
Rice bran oil	100.0	19.5	16.5	1.6	74.4	39.2	33.3	1.9	5.0	99
Safflower oil	100.0	9.4	6.4	2.5	86.2	11.9	73.3	1.0	0.8	140
Sesame oil	100.0	15.2	9.4	4.8	80.4	39.1	40.0	1.3	1.0	104
Soybean oil	100.0	15.0	10.7	3.9	80.6	22.8	50.8	7.0	1.2	133

[1] Includes α-linolenic acid (18:3, n–3) and long-chain essential fatty acids. – [2] Contains 35.1 g erucic acid (22:1, n–9). – [3] Contains 48.1 g erucic acid (22:1, n–9). – [4] Contains 0.2 g erucic acid (22:1, n–9).
See list of sources on page 92.

Sources for Appendix 1

Anderson, B.A., Kinsella, J.A. & Watt, B.K. Comprehensive evaluation of fatty acids in foods. Part 2. Beef products. *J. Amer. Diet. Assoc.*, 1975, 67:35.

Brignoli, C.A., Kinsella, J.A. & Weihrauch, J.L. Comprehensive evaluation of fatty acids in foods. Part 5. Unhydrogenated fats and oils. *J. Amer. Diet. Assoc.*, 1976, 68:224.

Exler, J., Kinsella, J.A. & Watt, B.K. Lipids and fatty acids of important fish: new data for nutrient tables. *J. Amer. Oil Chemists Soc.*, 1975, 52:154.

FAO/US Department of Health and Welfare. *Food composition table for use in East Asia*, 1972.

Fristrom, G.E., Steward, B.C., Weihrauch, J.L. & Posati, L.P. Comprehensive evaluation of fatty acids in foods. Part 4. Nuts, peanuts and soups. *J. Amer. Diet. Assoc.*, 1975, 67:351.

Posati, L.P., Kinsella, J.A. & Watt, B.K. Comprehensive evaluation of fatty acids in foods. Part 1. Dairy products. *J. Amer. Diet. Assoc.*, 1975, 66:483.

Posati, L.P., Kinsella, J.A. & Watt, B.K. Comprehensive evaluation of fatty acids in foods. Part 3. Eggs and egg products. *J. Amer. Diet. Assoc.*, 1975, 67:111.

Weihrauch, J.L., Kinsella, J.A. & Watt, B.K. Comprehensive evaluation of fatty acids in foods. Part 6. Cereal products. *J. Amer. Diet. Assoc.*, 1976, 68:335.

Home-made preparations as supplementary foods

Examples of possible formulas for food supplementation of two- to four-month-old infants based on easily available flours in different parts of the world are given below:

Formulas	Protein (%)	Invis. fat (%)	Fibre (%)	Water (%)	Energy		Added fat (g)	Energy in total mixture (kcal)
					(kcal/ 100 g)	(MJ/ 100 g)		
Maize flour + beans (ratio 2.2:1)	6.2	1.4	1.1	72	140	0.58	22	338/122 g
Wheat flour + legume (ratio 2:1)	5.9	1.4	1.1	70	168	0.70	21	357/121 g
Rice flour + soya (full fat; ratio 2.6:1)	3.9	1.3	0.5	70	101	0.42	12.5	214/112.5 g
Oatmeal + milk (ratio 2:1)	5.6	3.0	0.5	63	156	0.65	17	309/117 g

NOTE. It must be stressed that these mixtures are only examples of nutritional approaches under study and must therefore be carefully tested.

The first two mixtures provide equal amounts of protein from cereals and legumes; the third mixture provides two thirds of the protein from soya flour.

Assuming intakes of 600 ml of breast milk, the energy intake obtained when these mixtures are given in amounts to fulfil total nitrogen and essential amino acid safe levels of intake approaches the recommended energy requirements without exceeding them. (Note that the energy content of 150 g of the rice-soya mixture is equivalent to 100 g of the other mixtures.) The fats in these mixtures contribute 52–66% of the total energy and 32–34 kcal (0.13–0.14 MJ)/g of protein. Total energy is 55–60 kcal (0.23–0.25 MJ)/g of protein or 14–15 kcal (59–63 kJ)/kcal of protein. The net dietary protein energy % of the 600 ml of breast milk plus these supplementary feeds is above 7.5, which is satisfactory for small infants.

REFERENCES

1. PÉRISSÉ, J., SIZARET, F. & FRANÇOIS, P. (1969) *Nutr. Newsletter (FAO)*, 7(3): 1.
2. UNITED STATES DEPARTMENT OF HEALTH, EDUCATION AND WELFARE, PUBLIC HEALTH SERVICE (1966) *Nutrition Survey of Eastern Pakistan, March 1962– January 1964*. Bethesda, Md., National Institute of Health.
3. LEE, K.T., MORRISON, E.S., SCOTT, E.F. & GOODALE, F. (1962) *Circulation*, 26:600.
4. ROELS, O.A., TROUT, M. & DUJACQUIER, R. (1958) *J. Nutr.*, 65:115.
5. SALTIN, B. & HERMANSEN, L. (1967) *Nutrition and Physical Activity*, Blix, G. (ed.). Uppsala, Sweden, The Swedish Nutrition Foundation.
6. KARVONEN, N.J. (1967) *Nutrition and Physical Activity*, Blix, G. (ed.). Uppsala, Sweden, The Swedish Nutrition Foundation.
7. KARK, R.M., GROOME, R.R.M., CAWTHORPE, J., BELL, D.M., BRYAN, A., MACBETH, R.J., JOHNSON, R.E., CONSOLAZIO, F.C., POULIN, J.L., TAYLOR, F.H.L. & COGSWELL, F.C. (1948) *J. Appl. Physiol.*, 1:73.
8. CONSOLAZIO, F.C., SHAPIRO, R., MASTERSON, J.E. & McKINSIE, P.S.L. (1961) *J. Nutr.*, 73:126.
9. JOHNSON, R.E. & KARK, R.M. (1947) *Science* (N.Y.), 105:378.
10. YANG, M.U. & VAN ITALLIE, T.B. (1976) *J. Clin. Invest.*, 58:722.
11. JOINT FAO/WHO AD HOC EXPERT COMMITTEE ON ENERGY AND PROTEIN REQUIREMENTS (1973) FAO Nutrition Meeting Report Series No. 52, WHO Technical Report Series No. 522.
12. PASRICHA, S. (1958) *Indian J. Med. Res.*, 46:605.
13. WHO EXPERT COMMITTEE (1964) *Nutrition in pregnancy and lactation*. Geneva, WHO, Technical Report Series No. 302.
14. VENKATACHALAM, P.S. (1962) *Bull. Wld Hlth Org.*, 26:193.
15. VALYASEVI, A. (1964) *Second Far East Symposium on Nutrition*. 100 p. USA, Interdepartmental Committee on Nutrition for National Defense.
16. HYTTEN, P.E. & LEICHT, I. (1971) *The Physiology of Human Pregnancy*. Oxford, London, Blackwell Scientific Publications.
17. GHOSH, S. & DAGA, S. (1967) *J. Pediatrics*, 71:173.
18. LECHTIG, A., MARGEN, S., PARRELL, T., DELGADO, H., YARBROUGH, C.M., MARTORELL, R. & KLEIN, R.E. (1977) Low birth weight babies, world-wide incidence, economic costs and program needs. In *Perinatal Care in Developing Countries*. Engstrom, L. & Rooth, G. (eds). University of Uppsala, Perinatal Research Lab., Dept. Pediatrics.
19. STAHLIE, T.D. (1961) *J. Trop. Med. Hyg.*, 64:79.
20. MATA, L.J., URRUTIA, J.J., KRONMAL, A. & JOPLIN, C. (1975) *Amer. J. Dis. Child*, 129:561.
21. MEREDITH, H.V. (1970) *Human Biology*, 42:217.
22. CRAWFORD, M.A., HALL, B., LAWRENCE, B.M. & MUMHAMBO, A. (1976) *Current Med. Res. Opin.*, 4:33.
23. WATERLOW, J.C. & ALLEYNE, G.A.O. (1971) *Adv. Protein Chem.*, 25:117.
24. VITERI, F.E. & ARROYAVE, G. (1973) Protein-Calorie Malnutrition. In *Human Nutrition in Health and Disease*. Philadelphia, Lea and Febiger.

25. BENGOA, J.M. (1975) In *Protein-Calorie Malnutrition*, Olson, R.E. (ed.). New York, Academic Press.
26. LECHTIG, A., YARBROUGH, C., DELGADO, H., HABICHT, J.P., MARTORELL, R. & KLEIN, R.E. (1975) *Amer. J. Clin. Nutr.*, 28:1223.
27. GEBRE-MEDHIN, M.A., VAHLQUIST, A., HOFVANDER, Y., UPPSALL, L. & VAHLQUIST, B. (1976) *Amer. J. Clin. Nutr.*, 29:441.
28. BAILEY, K.V. (1965) *J. Trop. Pediat.*, 11:35.
29. THOMPSON, A.M. & BLACK, A.E. (1973) *Nutrition Aspects of Human Lactation*. Planning Meeting of Task Force on Collaborative Research on Breast Feeding. Geneva, WHO.
30. VITERI, F.E. & TORUN, B. (1976) *Bol. of Sanit. Panam.*, 78:58.
31. GOPALAN, C. & NARASINGA RAO, B.S. (1971) *Proc. Nutr. Soc. India*, 10:111.
32. FLORES, M., MENCHU, M.T., LARA, M.Y. & GUZMAN, M.A. (1970) *Archivos Latino-Americanos de Nutrición*, 22:255.
33. SUKHATME, P.V. (1970) *Brit. J. Nutr.*, 24:477.
33a. DEPARTMENT OF HEALTH AND SOCIAL SECURITY, UK (1976) *Present-day Infant Feeding Practices, Report No. 9.* London, Her Majesty's Stationery Office.
34. MATTSON, F.H. & VOLPENHEIN, R.A. (1962) *J. Biol. Chem.*, 237:53.
35. FILER, L.J., MATTSON, F.H. & FOMON, S.J. (1969) *J. Nutr.*, 99:293.
36. HADORN, B., ZOPPI, G., SCHMERLING, D.H., PRADER, A., McINTYRE, I. & ANDERSON, C.M. (1968) *J. Pediat.*, 73:39.
37. ZOPPI, G., ANDREOTTI, G., PAJNO-FERRARA, F., NJAI, D.M. & GABURRO, D. (1972) *Pediat. Res.*, 6:880.
38. LAVY, U., SILVERBERG, M. & DAVIDSON, M. (1971) *Pediat. Res.*, 5:387.
39. SIGNER, E., MURPHY, G.M., EDKINS, S. & ANDERSON, C.M. (1974) *Archs Dis. Child*, 49:174.
40. VITERI, F.E. & SCHNEIDER, R.E. (1974) *Med. Clin. North. Amer.*, 58:1487.
41. PARVATHI RAU, HANUMANTHA RAO, D., NADAMUNI NAIDU, A. & SWAMINATHAN, M.C. (1970) *Indian J. Nutr. Dietet.*, 7:337.
41a. VINODINI, R. & MAMMI, M.V.I. (1976) *J. Trop. Pediat. & Environ. Child Hlth*, 22:3.
42. DEUEL, H.J. & MOREHOUSE, M.G. (1946) *Adv. Carbohydrate Chem.*, 2:119.
43. NARASINGA RAO, B.S., VISWESWARA RAO, K. & NADAMUNI NAIDU, A. (1969) *Indian J. Nutr. Dietet.*, 6:238.
44. BURR, G.O. & BURR, M.M. (1929) *J. Biol. Chem.*, 82:345.
45. BURR, G.O. & BURR, M.M. (1930) *J. Biol. Chem.*, 86:587.
46. HANSEN, A.E. (1933) *Proc. Soc. Exptl Biol. Med.*, 31:160.
47. HANSEN, A.E. (1937) *Amer. J. Dis. Child*, 53:933.
48. HANSEN, A.E., KNOTT, E.M., WIESE, H.F., SHAPERMAN, E. & McQUARRIE, I. (1947) *Amer. J. Dis. Child*, 73:1.
49. HANSEN, A.E., WIESE, H.F., BIELSCHE, A.N., HAGGARD, M.E., ADAM, D.J.D. & DAVIS, H. (1963) *Pediatrics*, 31 (Suppl. I, Pt. 2):171.
50. COLLINS, F.D., SINCLAIR, A.J., ROYLE, J.P., COATS, D.A., MAYNARD, A.T. & LEONARD, R.F. (1971) *Nutr. Metabol.*, 13:150.
51. RIELLA, M.C., BROVIAC, J.W., WELLS, M. & SCRIBNER, B.H. (1975) *Ann. Internat. Med.*, 83:786.
52. STEGNIK, L.D., FREEMAN, J.B., WISPE, J. & CONNER, W.E. (1977) *Amer. J. Clin. Nutr.*, 30:388.
53. PRESS, M.P., HARTOP, J. & PROTTEY, C. (1974) *Lancet*, 2:597.
54. BÖHLES, H., BIEBER, M.A. & HEIRD, W.C. (1976) *Amer. J. Clin. Nutr.*, 29:398.
55. LAMPTEY, M.S. & WALKER, B.L. (1976) *J. Nutr.*, 106:86.
56. BENOLKEN, R.M., ANDERSON, R.E. & WHEELER, T.G. (1973) *Science* (N.Y.), 182:1253.

57. FIENNES, R.N.T.W., SINCLAIR, A.J. & CRAWFORD, M.A. (1973) *J. Med. Primatol.*, 2:155.
57a. LEE, D.J., ROEHM, J.N., YU, T.C. & SINNHUBER, R.O. (1967) *J. Nutr.*, 92:93.
58. HOUTSMULLER, U.M.T. (1975) In *The Role of Fats in Human Nutrition*, Vergroesen, A.J. (ed.). London, Academic Press.
58a. MOHRHAUER, H. & HOLMAN, R.T. (1963) *J. Lipid Res.*, 4:151.
58b. HASSAM, A.G., RIVERS, J.P.W. & CRAWFORD, M.A. (1977) *J. Nutr.*, 107:519.
59. HOLMAN, R.T. (1970) *Progress in the Chemistry of Fats and other Lipids*, 9:275, 555, 611.
60. HEGSTED, D.M., McGANDY, R.B., MYERS, M.L. & STARE, F.J. (1965) *Amer. J. Clin. Nutr.*, 17:128.
61. HORNSTRA, G. (1975) In *The Role of Fats in Human Nutrition*, Vergroesen, A.J. (ed.). London, Academic Press.
62. LANDS, W.E.M., BLANK, M.L., NUTTER, L.J. & PRIVETT, O.S. (1966) *Lipids*, 1:224.
63. HASSAN, H., HASHIM, S.A., VAN ITALLIE, T.B. & SEBRELL, W.H. (1966) *Amer. J. Clin. Nutr.*, 19:147.
64. CARROLL, K.K. & KHOR, H.T. (1971) *Lipids*, 6:415.
65. KING, M.M., BAILEY, D.M., GIBSON, D.D., PITHA, J.V. & McCAY, P.B. (1977) *Fed. Proc.*, 36:1148.
66. EDERER, F., LEREN, P., TURPEINEN, O. & FRANTZ, I.D., JR. (1971) *Lancet*, 2:203.
67. STURDEVANT, R.A.L., DAYTON, S. & PEARCE, M.L. (1972) *Abst. Cardiovascular Disease Epidemiology Conference*. American Health Association.
68. HOLMAN, R.T. (1977) Essential fatty acid deficiency in humans. In *Handbook of Nutrition and Foods*, Recheigl, M. (ed.). Cleveland, Ohio, C.R.C. Press.
69. HOLMAN, R.T. (1977) Essential fatty acid deficiency in animals. In *Handbook of Nutrition and Foods*, Recheigl, M. (ed.). Cleveland, Ohio, C.R.C. Press.
70. HOLMAN, R.T., CASTER, W.O. & WIESE, H.F. (1964) *Amer. J. Clin. Nutr.*, 14:70.
71. HOLMAN, R.T. (1978). In White, P.L. & Selvey, N. (eds), *Proc. West. Hemisphere Nutr. Congress*, Am. Med. Assoc.
72. BAGCHI, K., HALDER, K. & CHOWDHURY, S.D. (1959) *Amer. J. Clin. Nutr.*, 7:251.
73. KINGSBURY, K.J., BRITT, C., STOVALD, R., CHAPMAN, A., ANDERSON, J. & MORGAN, D.H. (1974) *Postgrad. Med. J.*, 50:425.
74. OLEGARD, R. & SVENNERHOLM, L. (1970) *Acta Pediat. Scand.*, 59:637.
75. CRAWFORD, M.A., HASSAM, A.G., WILLIAMS, G. & WHITEHOUSE, W.L. (1976) *Lancet*, 1:452.
75a. CRAWFORD, M.A., HASSAM, A.G., WILLIAMS, G. & WHITEHOUSE, W.L. (1977) In *Function and Biosynthesis of Lipids*, New York, Plenum Press.
76. APTE, S.V. & IYENGAR, L. (1972) *Brit. J. Nutr.*, 27:305.
76a. ROBERTSON, A.F. & SPRECHER, H. (1968) *Acta Pediat. Scand.*, Suppl. 183.
76b. WIDDOWSON, E.M. (1968) In *Biology of Gestation*, Asali, N.S. (ed.). New York, Academic Press.
76c. PAPE, E., STOLLEY, H. & DROESE, W. (1974) *Z. Kinderheilk.*, 116:269.
76d. ROUX, J.F., TAKEDA, Y. & GRIGORIAN, A. (1977) *Pediatrics*, 48:540.
77. CRAWFORD, M.A., LAURANCE, B.M., HALL, B., BERG-HANSEN, I. & MUNHAMBO, A. *Amer. J. Clin. Nutr.*
77a. DEPARTMENT OF HEALTH AND SOCIAL SECURITY, UK (1977) *Composition of mature milk*, Report on Health & Social Subjects No. 12. London, Her Majesty's Stationery Office.

78. HASSAM, A.G., SINCLAIR, A.J. & CRAWFORD, M.A. (1975) *Lipids*, 10:417.
79. RIVERS, J.P.W., SINCLAIR, A.J. & CRAWFORD, M.A. (1975) *Nature* (London), 258:171.
80. DeGOMEZ DUMM, I.M.T. & BRENNER, R.R. (1975) *Lipids*, 10:315.
81. COOTS, R.H. (1965) *J. Lipid Res.*, 6:494.
82. SINCLAIR, A.J. (1975) *Lipids*, 10:175.
83. HASSAM, A.G. & CRAWFORD, M.A. (1976) *J. Neurochem.*, 27:967.
84. SINCLAIR, A.J. & CRAWFORD, M.A. (1973) *Brit. J. Nutr.*, 29:127.
85. PAOLETTI, H. & GALLI, C. (1972) *Lipids, malnutrition and the developing brain.* CIBA Foundation Symposium. Amsterdam, Associated Scientific Publishers.
86. SUN, G.Y. & SUN, A.Y. (1974) *J. Neurochem.*, 22:15.
87. PIKAAR, N.A. & FERNANDEZ, J. (1966) *Amer. J. Clin. Nutr.*, 19:194.
88. SANDERS, T.A.B. & NAISMITH, D.J. (1976) *Proc. Nutr. Soc.*, 35:63A.
89. CRAWFORD, M.A., HASSAM, A.G. & HALL, B. (1977) *Nutr. Metabol.*, 21 (Suppl. 1):187.
90. OSBORN, C.R. (1963) *The Incubation Period of Coronary Thrombosis.* London, Butterworth.
91. SCHENDEL, H.H. & HANSEN, J.D.L. (1959) *South Afr. Med. J.*, 33:1005.
92. LAUW, M.E., DU PLESSIS, J.P. & VAN DEN BERG, A.S. (1969) *South Afr. Med. J.*, 43:1516.
93. CRAWFORD, M.A., HASSAM, A.G. & RIVERS, J.P.W. *Postgrad. Med. J.* (in press).
94. STRONG, J. (1972) *Atherosclerosis*, 16:193.
95. GORDON, T. (1957) *Pub. Health Rep., Washington*, 72:543.
95a. KALLNER, G. (1958) *Lancet*, 1:1155.
95b. ANTONOVSKY, A. (1971) *Isr. J. Med. Sci.*, 7:1578.
95c. EPSTEIN, F.H. (1965) *J. Chron. Dis.*, 18:735.
95d. KATO, H., TILLOTSON, J., MICHAMAN, M.Z., RHOADS, G.G. & HAMILTON, H.B. (1973) *Amer. J. Epidm.*, 97:372.
95e. DeHAAS, J.H. (1973) World Health Organization, WHO/CVD/73.1.
96. KANNEL, W.B. & DAWBER, T.D. (1972) *J. Pediat.*, 80:544.
97. FREDERICKSON, D.S. (1972) *Amer. J. Clin. Nutr.*, 25:221.
98. DE HAAS, J.H. (1973) *Heart Bull.*, 4:3.
99. HEYDEN, S. (1975) In *The Role of Fats in Human Nutrition*, Vergroesen, A.J. (ed.). London, Academic Press.
100. VERGROESEN, A.J. & GOTTENBOS, J.J. (1975) In *The Role of Fats in Human Nutrition*, Vergroesen, A.J. (ed.). London. Academic Press.
101. MCGANDY, R.B. & HEGSTED, D.M. (1975) In *The Role of Fats in Human Nutrition*, Vergroesen, A.J. (ed.). London, Academic Press.
102. NATIONAL HEART FOUNDATION OF AUSTRALIA (1974) *Med. J. Aust.*, 1:575.
103. FREDERICKSON, D.S. (1972) *Mod. Concepts Cardiovascular Dis.*, 41:31.
104. FREDERICKSON, D.S. & LEVY, R.J. (1972) *The Metabolic Basis of Inherited Disease.* New York, McGraw-Hill.
105. GLUECK, C.J. & TSANG, R.C. (1972) *Amer. J. Clin. Nutr.*, 25:224.
106. HAUST, M.D. (1970) *Atherosclerosis.* Berlin, Springer Verlag.
107. WESSLER, A. (1974) *J. Amer. Med. Assoc.*, 228:757.
108. HORNSTRA, G. (1975) In *The Role of Fats in Human Nutrition*, Vergroesen, A.J. (ed.). London, Academic Press.
109. MIETTINEN, M., TURPEINEN, O., KARVONEN, M.J., ELUOSO, R. & PAAVILAINEN, E. (1972) *Lancet*, 1:835.
110. HORNSTRA, G., LEWIS, B., CHAIT, A., TURPEINEN, O., KARVONEN, J.J. & VERGROESEN, A.J. (1973) *Lancet*, 1:1155.

111. FLEISCHMAN, A.I., JUSTICE, D., BIERENBAUM, M.L., STIER, A. & SULLIVAN, A. (1975) *J. Nutr.*, 105:1286.
112. O.BRIEN, J.R., ETHERINGTON, M.D. & JAMIESON, S. (1976) *Lancet*, 1:878.
113. DAWBER, T.R., KANNELL, A., KAGAN, A., DONABEDIAN, R.K., McNAMARA, P.M. & PEARSON, G. (1967) In *The Epidemiology of Hypertension.*, Stamler, Stamler and Pulman (eds). New York, Grune & Stratton.
114. TRIEBE, G., BLOCK, H. & FURSTER, W. (1976) *Acta Biol. Med. Germ.*, 35:1223.
115. TEN HOOR, F. & VAN DE GRAAF, H.M. *Nutr. Metabol.* (in press)
116. VANE, J.B. (1971) *Nature (New Biol.)*, 231:232.
117. LEE, J.B. (1976) *Amer. J. Med.*, 61:681.
118. MARKOV, H.M. (1976) *Acta Biol. Med. Germ.*, 35:1201.
119. SOMOVA, L. (1976) *Acta Biol. Med. Germ.*, 35:1207.
120. IACONO, J.M., MARSHALL, H.W., DOUGHERTY, R.M., WHEELER, M.A., MACKIN, J.F. & CANARY, J.J. (1975) *Prevent. Med.*, 4:426.
121. COMBERG, H.U., HEYDEN, S., VERGROESEN, A.J. & FLEISCHMAN, A.I. (1978) *Acta Biol. Med. Germ.* (in press)
122. KANNEL, W.B. & GORDON, T. (1975) *Recent Advances in Obesity Research*, 1:14.
123. VAN STRATUM, P., LUSSENBURG, R.N., VAN WEZEL, L.A., VERGROESEN, A.J. & CREMER, H.D. (1978) *Amer. J. Clin. Nutr.*, 31:206.
124. ANON. (1971) *Lancet*, 1:583.
125. HOUTSMULLER, A.J. (1975) In *The Role of Fats in Human Nutrition*, Vergroesen, A.J. (ed). London, Academic Press.
126. FELIG, P. (1975) In *Diabetes Mellitus*, Sussman, K.E. & Metz, R.T.S. (eds). New York, American Diabetic Association.
127. STOUT, R.W. (1977) *Atherosclerosis*, 27:1.
128. METZ, R.J.S. (1975) In *Diabetes Mellitus*, Sussman, K.E. & METZ, R.T.S. (eds). New York, American Diabetic Association.
129. WEST, K.M. (1975) In *Diabetes Mellitus*, Sussman, K.E. & Metz, R.T.S. (eds). New York, American Diabetic Association.
130. JOSLIN, E.P. & WHITE, P. (1965) *Med. Clin. North. Amer.*, 49:905.
131. WESSELS, M., GRIES, F.A., IRMCHER, K., LIEBERMEISTER, H., BUCHENAU, H. & VIEHWEGER, J. (1970) *Deut. Med. Wschr.*, 95:382.
132. FANCONI, G. (1955) *Schweiz. Med. Wschr.*, 85:75.
132a. NOLEN, G.A., ALEXANDER, J.C. & ARTMAN, N.R. (1967) *J. Nutr.*, 93:337.
132b. ALFIN-SLATER, R.B., WELLS, P. & AFTERGOOD, L. (1973) *J. Amer. Oil Chemists Soc.*, 50:479.
132c. ROWSELL, H.C., DOWNIE, H.G. & MUSTARD, J.F. (1958) *Canad. Med. J.*, 79:647.
132d. ALFIN-SLATER, R.B., AFTERGOOD, L., HANSEN, H., MORRIS, R.S., MELNICK, D. & GOODING, C.M. (1966) *J. Amer. Oil Chemists Soc.*, 43:110.
133. PHELPS, R.A., SHENSTONE, F.S., KEMMERER, A.R. & EVANS, R.J. (1965) *Poultry Sci.*, 44:358.
134. TATTRIE, N.H. & YAGUCHI, M. (1973) *Can. Inst. Food Sci. Technol. J.*, 6:289.
135. ANDREWS, J.S., GRIFFITH, W.H., MEED, J.F. & STEIN, R.A. (1960) *J. Nutr.*, 70:199.
136. PARSONS, A.M. (1970) *Progr. Chem. Fats Lipids*, 11:245.
137. ROST, H.E. (1976) *Chem. and Ind.*, 17 July, p. 612.
138. NATIONAL INSTITUTE OF NUTRITION (1976) *Annual Report*. Hyderabad, Indian Council of Medical Research.
139. AAES-JØRGENSEN, E. (1972) Nutritional value of rapeseed oil. In *Rapeseed*, Applequist, L.A. & Ohlson, R. (eds). Amsterdam, Elsevier Publishing Co.

140. VLES, R.O. (1975) In *The Role of Fats in Human Nutrition*, Vergroesen, A.J. (ed). London, Academic Press.
141. BEARE-ROGERS, J.L. (1977) *Progress in Chemistry of Fats and Other Lipids*, 15:29.
142. WAGNER, H., SEELIG, E. & BERNHARD, K. (1956) Z. *Physiol. Chem.*, 306:96.
143. WAGNER, H., SEELIG, E. & BERNHARD, K. (1958) Z. *Physiol. Chem.*, 312:104.
144. WALKER, B.L., ATKINSON, S.M., ZEHALUK, C.M. & MACKEY, M.G. (1972) *Comp. Biochem. Physiol.*, 42B:619.
145. WALKER, B.L., LALL, S.P., SLINGER, S.J. & BAYLEY, H.S. (1970) *Marketing rapeseed and rapeseed products. Proc. Int. Conf. Sci. Technol. Can.*, 377.
146. CRAIG, B.M., YOUNGS, C.G., BEARE, J.L. & CAMPBELL, J.A. (1963) *Can. J. Biochem. Physiol.*, 41:43.
147. KRAMER, J.G.K., MAHADEVAN, S., HUNT, J.R., SAUER, F.D., CORNER, A.H. & CHARLTON, K.M. (1973) *J. Nutr.*, 103:1696.
148. KRAMER, M. (1973) *Die Nahrung*, 17:643.
149. WALKER, B.L. (1972) *Can. J. Anim. Sci.*, 52:713.
150. BERNHARD, K., LINDLAR, F. & WAGNER, H. (1960) Z. *Ernährungswiss.*, 1:48.
151. BEARE, J.L. (1961) *Can. J. Biochem. Physiol.*, 39:1855.
152. ROCQUELIN, G.C.R. (1972) *C.R. hebd. séances*, 274:592. Paris, Acad. Sci.
153. BLOMSTRAND, R. & SVENSSON, L. (1975) *Acta Medica Scand.*, Suppl. 585:51.
154. CARROLL, K.K. (1953) *J. Biol. Chem.*, 200:287.
155. CARROLL, K.K. (1962) *Can. J. Biochem. Physiol.*, 40:1115.
156. CARROLL, K.K. & NOBLE, R.L. (1952) *Endocrinology*, 51:476.
157. BEARE, J.L., GREGORY, E.R.W., SMITH, D.M. & CAMPBELL, J.A. (1961) *Can. J. Biochem. Physiol.*, 39:195.
158. CARROLL, K.K. (1951) *Endocrinology*, 48:101.
159. ABDELLATIF, A.M.M. & VLES, R.O. (1970) *Nutr. Metabol.*, 12:285.
160. ABDELLATIF, A.M.M. & VLES, R.O. (1970) *Marketing rapeseed and rapeseed products. Proc. Int. Conf. Sci. Technol. Can.*, 423.
161. ABDELLATIF, A.M.M. & VLES, R.O. (1971) *Voeding*, 32:602.
162. WALKER, B.L. & CARNEY, J.A. (1971) *Lipids*, 6:797.
163. BEARE, J.L., MURRAY, T.K., McLAUGHLAN, J.M. & CAMPBELL, J.A. (1963) *J. Nutr.*, 80:157.
164. BEARE-ROGERS, J.L. (1972) *The 11th World Congress of the International Society for Fat Research. Abstracts of papers*, Göteborg.
165. CARROLL, K.K. & NOBLE, R.L. (1957) *Can. J. Biochem. Physiol.*, 35:1093.
166. BEARE, J.L., GREGORY, E.R.W. & CAMPBELL, J.A. (1959) *Can. J. Biochem. Physiol.*, 37:1191.
167. ROCQUELIN, G., MARTIN, B. & CLUZAN, R. (1970) *Marketing rapeseed and rapeseed products. Proc. Int. Conf. Sci. Technol. Can.*, 405.
168. THOMASSON, H.J. (1955) *J. Nutr.*, 57:17.
169. THOMASSON, H.J., GOTTENBOS, J.J., VAN PIJPEN, P.L. & VLES, R.O. (1967) *Int. Symp. Chem. Technol. Rapeseed and Other Cruciferae Oils, Poland*, 381.
170. ABDELLATIF, A.M.M. & VLES, R.O. (1970) *Nutr. Metabol.*, 12:296.
171. VLES, R.O. & ABDELLATIF, A.M.M. (1970) *Marketing rapeseed and rapeseed products. Proc. Int. Conf. Sci. Technol. Can.*, 435.
172. ABDELLATIF, A.M.M. & VLES, R.O. (1971) *Nutr. Metabol.*, 13:65.
173. ABDELLATIF, A.M.M., STARRENBURG, A. & VLES, R.O. (1972) *Nutr. Metabol.*, 14:17.
174. BERGLUND, F. (1975) *Acta Medica Scand.*, Suppl. 585.
175. CARROLL, K.K. (1957) *Proc. Soc. Exp. Biol. Med.*, 94:202.

176. HOUTSMULLER, U.M.T., STRUIJK, C.B. & VAN DER BEEK, A. (1970) *Biochim. Biophys. Acta.*, 218:564.
177. BEARE-ROGERS, J.L., NERA, E.A. & HEGGTVEIT, H.A. (1971) *Can. Inst. Food Technol. J.*, 4:120.
178. ABDELLATIF, A.M.M. & VLES, R.O. (1973) *Nutr. Metabol.*, 15:219.
179. BEARE-ROGERS, J.L. (1970) *Marketing rapeseed and rapeseed products.* Proc. Int. Conf. Sci. Technol. Can., 450.
180. BEARE-ROGERS, J.L. & NERA, E.A. (1972) *Comp. Biochem. Physiol.*, 41B:793.
181. BEARE-ROGERS, J.L., NERA, E.A. & CRAIG, B.M. (1972) *Lipids*, 7:548.
182. BEARE-ROGERS, J.L., NERA, E.A. & CRAIG, B.M. (1972) *Lipids*, 7:46.
183. CHRISTOPHERSEN, B.O. & BREMER, J. (1972) *FEBS Lett.*, 23:230.
184. CHRISTOPHERSEN, B.O. & BREMER, J. (1972) *Biochim. Biophys. Acta*, 280:506.
185. GUMPEN, S.A. & NORUM, K.R. (1973) *Biochim. Biophys. Acta*, 316:48.
186. ENGFELDT, B. & BRUNIUS, E. (1975) *Acta Medica Scand.* Suppl. 585:27.
187. ENGFELDT, B. & BRUNIUS, E. (1975) *Acta Medica Scand.* Suppl. 585:15.
188. TEN HOOR, F., VAN DE GRAAF, H.M. & VERGROESEN, A. (1973) *Recent Advances in Studies on Cardiac Structure and Metabolism*, 3:59.
189. MACDONALD, B. (1974) *Proc. 4th Int. Conf. Rapeseed.* Giessen, Germany, F.R.
190. DEUEL, H.J., CHENG, A.L.S. & MOREHOUSE, M.G. (1948) *J. Nutr.*, 35:295.
191. HOLMES, A.D. (1918) *U.S. Dept. Agr. Bull.*, 687.
192. SWARTTOUW, M.A. (1974) *Biochim. Biophys. Acta*, 337:13.
193. CHRISTIANSEN, R.Z., CHRISTOPHERSEN, B.O. & BREMER, J. (1972) *Biochim. Biophys. Acta*, 280:506.
194. CHRISTIANSEN, R.Z., CHRISTOPHERSEN, B.O. & BREMER, J. (1975) *Biochim. Biophys. Acta*, 388:402.
195. CHRISTIANSEN, R.Z., CHRISTOPHERSEN, B.O. & BREMER, J. (1977) *Biochim. Biophys. Acta*, 487:28.
196. CRAIG, B.M. & BEARE, J.L. (1968) *Can. Inst. Food Techn. J.*, 1:64.
196a. THOMASSON, H.J. & BOLDINGH, J. (1955) *J. Nutr.*, 56:469.
197. ROCQUELIN, G. & CLUZAN, R. (1968) *Ann. Biol. Anim. Biochem. Biophys.*, 8:395.
198. ROCQUELIN, G., SERGIEL, J.P., ASTORG, P.O., NITON, G., VODOVAR, N., CLUZAN, R. & LEVILLEIN, R. (1974) *Proc. 4th Int. Conf. Rapeseed.* Giessen, Germany, F.R.
199. LAPOUS, D., KETEVI, P. & LORIETTE, C. (1974) *Ann. Biol. Anim. Biochem. Biophys.*, 14:689.
200. HULAN, H.W., KRAMER, J.K.G., MAHADEVAN, S. & SAUER, F.D. (1976) *Lipids*, 11:9.
201. BEARE-ROGERS, J.L., NERA, E.A. & HEGGTVEIT, H.A. (1974) *Nutr. Metabol.*, 17:213.
202. VLES, R.O., BIJSTER, G.M., KLEINEKOORT, J.S.W., TIMMER, W.G. & ZAALBERG, J. (1976) *Fette, Seifen, Anstrichmittel 78*, 3:128.
203. BEARE-ROGERS, J.L. (1977) *Symp. Rapeseed Oil, Meal and By-product Utilization.* Vancouver, Canada.
204. ABDELLATIF, A.M.M. & VLES, R.O. (1973) *Poult. Sci.*, 52:1932.
204a. LEVILLAIN, R., VEDOVAR, N., FLANZY, J., CLUZAN, R. (1972) *C.R. Soc. Biol.*, 12:1633.
204b. LOEW, F.M. *et al.* (1977) *Fisheries and Marine Service Technical Report*, 719:38. Halifax, Canadian Dept. of the Environment.
205. UTNE, F., NJAA, L.R., BRAEKKAN, O.R., LAMBERTSEN, G. & JULSHAMM, K. (1977) *Fisk. Dir. Ser. Ernaering*, 1:23.

206. ALAVAIKKO, M., HIRVONEN, J. & RÄSÄNEN, O. (1970) *Acta Path. Microbiol. Scand.*, Section A, 78:458.
207. BANG, H.O., DYERBERG, J. & HJØRNE, N. (1976) *Acta Med. Scand.*, 200:69.
208. DYERBERG, J., BANG, H.O. & HJØRNE, N. (1977) *Dan. Med. Bull.*, 24:52.
209. McKINNEY, B. (1974) *Pathology of the Cardiomyopathies*. London, Butterworth.
210. ACKMAN, R.G. (1974) *Lipids*, 9:1032.
211. ASTORG, P.O. & CLUZAN, R. (1976) *Ann. Nutr. Aliment.*, 30:581.
212. ASTORG, P.O. & ROCQUELIN, G. (1973) *C.R. hebd. séances*, 277:797. Paris, Acad. Sci.
213. SVAAR, H. & LANGMARK, F.T. (1974) *Inserm, Colloque de Synthèse, Série Action Thématique*, 2:329.
214. SVAAR, H., LANGMARK, F.T., LAMBERTSEN, G. & OPSTVEDT. *J. Acta Path. Microbiol. Scand.* (in press)
215. LOEW, F.M., SCHIEFER, B., FORSYTH, G.W., OLFERT, E.D., LAXDAL, V. & ACKMAN, R.G. (1977) *Fisheries and Marine Service Technical Report*, 719:73.
216. SCHLENK, H. (1972) *Fed. Proc.*, 31:1430.
217. BERNARDINI, M.P., BONIFORTI, L., SALVATI, S., SERLUPI, C.G., SPADONI, M.A., TAGLIAMONTE, B. & TOMASSI, G. (1976) *Nutr. Rep. Int.*, 14:405.
218. PROTEIN-CALORIE ADVISORY GROUP (1976) *Proceedings of the Symposium on Single Cell Proteins for Animal Feeding*. Brussels.
219. CRAWFORD, M.A., GALE, M.M., WOODFORD, M.W. & CASPERD, N.M. (1970) *Int. J. Biochem.*, 1:295.
220. CRAWFORD, M.A. (1975) *Proc. III Wld Cong. Animal Production, Melbourne*, Reid, E.L. (ed.). Sydney, University Press.
221. VERGROESEN, A.J. Personal communication.
222. BLAXTER, K.L. (1962) *The Energy Metabolism of Ruminants*. London, Hutchinson Scientific and Technical Publishers.
223. BLACK, J.L., GRAHAM, N.M.C. & FAICHNEY, G.J. (1976) In *Reviews of Rural Science*, 2:161. Sutherland, T.M., McWilliam, J.R. & Leng, R.A. (eds). Armidah, University of New England.
224. LEDGER, H.P. (1968) *Symposium Zool. Soc. Lond.*, 21:289.
225. CRAWFORD, M.A., GALE, M.M. & WOODFORD, M.H. (1970) *Intern. J. Biochem.*, 1:654.
225a. HUBBARD, A.W. & POCKLINGTON, W.D. (1968) *J. Sci. Fd Agric.*, 19:571.
226. SCOTT, T.W., COOK, L.J., FERGUSON, K.A., McDONALD, I.W., BUCHANAN, R.A. & LOFTUS HILLS, G. (1970) *Aust. J. Sci.*, 32:291.
227. CONNOLLY, J.F. (1974) *Farm Food Res.*, 512:41.

SOCIAL SCIENCE LIBRARY

Oxford University Library Services
Manor Road
Oxford OX1 3UQ
Tel: (2)71093 (enquiries and renewals)
http://www.ssl.ox.ac.uk

This is a NORMAL LOAN item.

We will email you a reminder before this item is due.

Please see http://www.ssl.ox.ac.uk/lending.html
for details on:

- loan policies; these are also displayed on the notice boards and in our library guide.

- how to check when your books are due back.

- how to renew your books, including information on the maximum number of renewals.
  Items may be renewed if not reserved by another reader. Items must be renewed before the library closes on the due date.

- level of fines; fines are charged on overdue books.

Please note that this item may be recalled during Term.